T0372916

Harnessing Hope in Managing Chronic Illness

Harnessing hope is fundamental to adapting to a chronic illness or palliative illness, and this fascinating book provides a new framework that will enable physiotherapists and other healthcare professionals to engage with patients to create better interactions and outcomes for rehabilitation.

Based on extensive research into how patients express their experiences, it identifies those factors that influence how hope can be used to benefit an interaction. It also considers central questions to illustrate how interactions can be psychologically mapped to assess emotions, adjustment, and hope. The book then features practical guidance on how to integrate the idea of hope into therapeutic conversations with patients, fostering acceptance and adaptation to the present, and looking towards the future.

This book will interest any practitioner working with patients experiencing chronic pain or palliative illness, as well as students across physiotherapy, occupational therapy, and community nursing. It may also interest any general readers facing challenges around trauma or loss.

Dr Andrew Soundy received his PhD from the University of Exeter, UK, in 2006. His interest in mental health during this time was ignited by a passion around the experiences of individuals with schizophrenia. He undertook his post-doctoral research at the University of Birmingham in 2005, with a focus on health psychology and physical activity. He began research on the concept of hope in 2009. His research has focused on chronic and palliative illness populations, often with a focus on neurological conditions. This work considers the experiences and perspectives of patients, caregivers, and healthcare professionals. The work has often been qualitative in nature, theory generating, and from 2019 onwards very applied to the pragmatic interactions of healthcare professionals. One of his greatest ambitions is to help healthcare professionals create more hopeful interactions with patients. To date, he has published over 120 articles and has experience working with global research groups and global organisations such as the World Health Organisation. His current research is devoted to improving patient interactions and training universities and NHS Trusts across the UK. This current book can summarise some of this focus and bring together essential developments from scholars studying the concept of hope and interactions from across the globe.

Harnessing Hope in Managing Chronic Illness

A Guide to Therapeutic Rehabilitation

Andrew Soundy

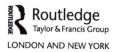

Routledge
Taylor & Francis Group

LONDON AND NEW YORK

First published 2025
by Routledge
4 Park Square, Milton Park, Abingdon, Oxon OX14 4RN

and by Routledge
605 Third Avenue, New York, NY 10158

Routledge is an imprint of the Taylor & Francis Group, an informa business

© 2025 Andrew Soundy

British Library Cataloguing-in-Publication Data
A catalogue record for this book is available from the British Library

ISBN: 978-1-032-73826-0 (hbk)
ISBN: 978-1-032-73828-4 (pbk)
ISBN: 978-1-003-46616-1 (ebk)

DOI: 10.4324/9781003466161

Typeset in Times New Roman
by Apex CoVantage, LLC

During the most difficult and uncertain times in my life, I have found a firm foundation from my faith in Jesus. This book is dedicated to Him.

Contents

Preface

A lot of my past research has focused on chronic illnesses and the idea of hope and the ability to look forward. This research area is currently flourishing, but I felt the breath of understanding about this area was not yet fully utilised in practice to support people during times of suffering. During times of distress and suffering, the ability to look forward may seem impossible. Whilst someone may, in the right conditions, be motivated and energised to look forward, suffering in life, including experiences of illness, grief, loss of relationships, roles, or jobs, can place a big challenge on anyone wanting a similar view. Such moments may be complicated by additional stresses and challenges; people at such a time may lack energy; they may feel captive to their situation rather than being hopeful for the future, a hope for survival or a hope for the suffering to end may be more possible and may be all that can be seen. Another hope may appear for a quick fix or an end to the situation that has caused suffering. However, if the change does not come and nothing seems hopeful, an individual can feel and embody an experience of being completely broken and overwhelmed, without any perception of control or energy. This may be because of the different circumstances that have come at once or the depth and impact of a particular circumstance. At such a time, what may be possible is the ability not to give up, and that may take all the energy and effort that an individual has. Further to this, such situations may not pass quickly, and they may last for years. However, I believe that all people can change and that it is possible, even in such circumstances, to regain motivation and energy. That is not to say such experiences are forgotten; situations and circumstances we live through can become scars from the past, or like a mental pit or trap that can be fallen into. From my own experience, such instances reduce across time and can become less intensive or effective in stopping you, but the mental trap may not easily be forgotten.

I believe in the potential for people to change, and I believe that as a part of supporting people to access that potential, healthcare professionals need to have the communication tools which help them understand the challenges faced by people quickly and in a meaningful way. An important goal of the work is to reduce suffering and help people find meaning and motivation. The work has been developed to harness hope by focusing on a simple psychological assessment through listening and asking specific questions, which provide a map of how the individual is adapting to a challenge they are facing. What makes this work unique is how it draws on specific hope literature to understand and support challenges and difficulties faced by people with chronic illness. This book was written as a way to consider and develop hope-centred interactions. The work is aimed at generating meaningful interactions that consider if a difficulty or challenge requires further understanding. The work also highlights the importance of, and provides a way to capture essential concepts relating to psycholgoical and emotional adaptation as well as hope in relation to a named difficulty.

The main tool described in later chapters is named the model of emotions, adaptation, and hope (MEAH). The book provides some practical application of using the concepts in specific ways to aid conversations rather than providing a critical overview of the concepts. The term model may be misleading for readers in terms of comparing the work to other models of therapies. I wouldn't describe this work as therapy but as something to enhance understanding of how individuals are managing. The work is aimed at helping understand the process of adaptation and being able to support hope-centred interactions. The goal of many therapies is to change thoughts and behaviour, and they are often underlined by principles or conditions and often require a process of learning before application. Rather than focusing on where or how a patient needs to change, this work looks to help develop a need to focus on adaptation, hope and energy, and feelings to develop a good understanding around how an individual is responding to a challenge and then, if needed, further explore the situation for factors which may influence that and the possibility of creating goals. This process is short and enables meaningful conversations to be developed where an individual feels heard. The application of the work will help increase hope and trust in the practitioner as well as empower the individual to consider their future.

The psycho-therapeutic benefit for patients that has been identified when applying this work results from being heard and understood. The benefit for practitioners has been reported as feeling more able to navigate difficult interactions. The development of the work has been within physiotherapy education, and the work has demonstrated that there can be an efficient, pragmatic way of identifying people who are in circumstances, which make feeling motivated and ready to progress with therapy very difficult or impossible. One of the guiding principles of the work is that a tool is developed that is easy to learn and can be applied in a single session. My research has shown that this can be learned quickly (<50 minutes of e-training) and delivered during a single short interaction. As part of the training now provided to physiotherapists across the UK, the work is used in different ways, including as (a) a screening tool (< 30 seconds), (b) a very brief therapy tool (applied in 10 minutes), or (c) an extended therapy tool where the understanding is considered in more depth

and a goal is developed (applied in 30 minutes). The purpose of the main tool
that is presented is to help start an interaction, create trust, and establish a relationship, where hope can flourish. The purpose of the extended version is to
use a fuller understanding of hope and the factors that influence hope to help
guide a meaningful conversation towards an identified goal. Where a goal is
not identified, benefit has still been found. Finally, it is important to note that
whilst the book is focused on chronic illness, the main model developed cer-
tainly has a broader application to consider how hope can be created and how
psychological and emotional adaptation is understood.

1 Introduction

How is hope defined?

Marcel (1951) states hope is the act by which the temptation to despair is overcome. Prusyer (1963) specifically associated hope with a response to stress or a response to the tragedy associated with an illness. Put in another way, Lazarus (1999) identifies that hope is a condition which results from life circumstances which are unsatisfactory, and this could include facing circumstances which are perceived as threatening, damaging, or depriving. Cutcliffe and Herth (2002) identify the opposite to hope is hopeless. They note that two other words originate from the same Latin root as hopelessness including despair and desperation. Across many review-based studies, hope was found to be in contrast or the opposite of despair, depression, hopelessness, fear, and anxiety (Olsman, 2021). Currently, there appears to be no universal definition of hope (de Graaf, 2016), and authors (Herrestad et al., 2014) have identified that there is limited value in establishing one. Smith (2008) identifies philosophers such as Hobbes (1968), Locke (1975), and Hume (1978) share an understanding that hope is related to obtaining something that will probably occur. From a religious perspective, Pinsent (2020) identifies that Aquinas situates hope as a theological virtual, which is associated with the seeking out of something that is good, and that hope belongs to the individual who has it, and that hope has its correct grounding in God and is associated with the salvation of man. More recent definitions of hope identify that it has a spiritual dimension (Scioli et al., 2011).

All the above definitions of hope highlight feelings as a component of hope and identify that what is hoped for is agreeable and wanted by that individual. More recent studies have identified hope as a framework or identified components which make up hope (DuFault & Martocchio, 1985; Hammer et al., 2009; Hasse et al., 1992; Morse & Doberneck, 1995; Owen, 1989; Reder & Serwint, 2009; Schrank et al., 2010). The most consistent component across all studies was that hope was associated with looking forward towards a future that was good or positive. Schrank et al. (2010) identified that what

DOI: 10.4324/9781003466161-1

is hoped for can be stimulated by a negative condition in the present. Other authors caveat this position, by identifying that what is hoped for should be considered being possible to achieve (DuFault & Martocchio, 1985) or that possibility exists for success (Hammer et al., 2009). Authors note that hope can be experienced with a certain level of uncertainty or unease (Hasse et al., 1992), and being able to look forward is associated with past successful coping efforts (Schrank et al., 2010). Five studies (Hasse et al., 1992; Hammer et al., 2009; Morse & Doberneck, 1995; Reder & Serwint, 2009; Schrank et al., 2010) include the view that hope is associated with identifying goals. Three studies (DuFault & Martocchio, 1985; Morse & Doberneck, 1995; Owen, 1989) identified that what is hoped for is regarded as meaningful to the individual. Three studies (Hammer et al., 2009; Morse & Doberneck, 1995; Reder & Serwint, 2009) identify the importance of understanding threats to hope and being able to meet the demands faced by the threat. Other references to hope were represented by fewer studies. This included, hope as a way of behaving and thinking (Farren et al., 1995; Stephenson, 1991), a way of being (Hammer et al., 2009) or a feeling, an emotion (Farren et al., 1995; Scioli et al., 2011; Stephenson, 1991), or an energised state (Hasse et al., 1992). Like emotions, hope is considered dynamic and variable (Schrank et al., 2010).

Colla et al. (2022) state that most literature considering hope defines it as a unidimensional construct which is associated with a perception that goals can be met. Achieving goals links to the doing dimension of hope and onto satisfaction (Hammer et al., 2009). This form of hope is most often used to establish the association of hope with other important constructs, for instance well-being or quality of life (Murphy, 2023). The origins of looking at hope as a unidimensional construct can be seen in research from the 1960s. For instance, Stotland (1969) defined hope as an expectation which is greater than zero of achieving a goal. Hope has been considered a driving force which enables goal-directed behaviour (French, 1952; Pruyser, 1963, Snyder et al., 1991). Such behaviour was identified as helping to reduce mental tension or worry about a situation and instead allowed the individual to identify something which is wished for and positive (French, 1952; Pruyser, 1986). An important progress around the association between hope and goals was made by the author Snyder (Snyder et al., 1991). Snyder et al. (1991) introduce the idea that two specific ingredients are needed for the process of hope to occur. The first ingredient is for a sense of determination (agency) which is goal directed. The second ingredient is for an understanding of the planning (pathways) needed to meet those goals. As he states, *"hope is defined as a positive motivational state that is based on interactively derived sense of successful (a) agency (goals directed energy), and (b) pathways (planning to meet goals)"* (Synder et al., 1991, p. 287). (Marques & Lopez, 2017) make two important observations about agency and pathways. First is that the determination to act (agency) increases as a desired future gets closer,

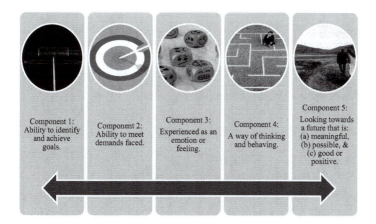

Figure 1.1 The major components of hope as identified across studies.

and second is that pathway thinking requires the ability to imagine different ways to achieve goals and is positively associated with curiosity and creativity in people. Figure 1.1 provides a visual of the major components of hope when considered a framework across studies.

Whilst focus on goals and Snyder's work is extremely valuable and useable within rehabilitation, this view of hope misses the importance of the other elements of hope identified in Figure 1.1. For instance, it may be that an individual does not believe they can meet a threat or the demands they face, or that their past experiences and current situation leave them with little energy and/or ability to look forward to a meaningful future. Further to this there is a tension between the reduction in mental tension created by feeling hope and looking forward, and the extent to which the experience is more dominated by uncertainty or a feeling of unease which may prevent goals being identified. Further understanding of the various component of hope may be needed to understand this and create the conditions to allow goals to be utilised more effectively. This could include an assessment of current emotions and perceived ability to meet threats to hope or demands that are faced (Soundy et al., 2016b). I have developed a focus on the importance of understanding emotions and psychological adaptation to understand challenges (Soundy, 2018), and the factors which support hope (Soundy et al., 2014c) before goals are created to harness hope (Soundy et al., 2023). Further to this, two aspects of my work need to be mentioned to give greater context to supporting hope. The first is the need to understand the levels of hope. This includes hoping for suffering to stop, considering the impact of the disease on an individual's social identities and roles, meaningful activities and relationships as well as the ability to accept and understand this impact, especially if the change is experienced as shock (Soundy et al., 2014a, 2014b). The second is to understand the different factors related to hope and appreciate the different levels of hope (Soundy et al., 2014c).

The difference between hope and related concepts

Before I continue, it is important that hope and other related concepts are distinguished. Several concepts have been identified as similar or sharing properties with hope. Rand (2018) identifies differences in hope from optimism and self-efficacy. Optimism reflects a general expectancy that good rather than bad things will happen. This type of optimism is also referred to as dispositional optimism (Dosedlová et al., 2016). It differs from hope as it is not self-focused and does not reflect any perceived influence of the individual on the outcome identified (Rand, 2018). Self-efficacy is identified and associated with the belief an individual has in their ability to succeed in performing a behaviour; however, whilst hope includes a factor of willpower, self-efficacy is identified as situation specific rather than reflecting more of a trait like nature (Rand, 2018). Wiles et al. (2008) identify the importance of understanding particularised hopes (hopes which are focused on a goal), and this type of hope is then sub-divided by Wiles et al. (2008) to represent hope as an expectation or as a wish. Hope as an expectation is considered expecting an outcome to occur because it is likely to happen. Expectation has also been considered response expectancy. Response expectancies are defined as the anticipation of the nonvolitional reactions to situations and behaviours that an individual has (David et al., 2004).

Why being hopeful is important?

Hope has been identified as a resource which is powerful for life and can help restore one's being (Holdcraft & Williamson, 1991). Conversely, the absence of hope can make life very bleak because without it there is no reason to live (Penz & Duggleby, 2011). Hope is vital at times of crisis or stress (Conway et al., 2017), and those people who are more hopeful are more able to overcome situations of extreme distress (Javier-Aliga et al., 2022). Indeed, it has long been considered that having hope has been associated with healing and should be considered within treatment following illness (Miller, 2007; Synder et al., 1991). Hope has been associated with other outcomes too. For instance, better academic achievements, happiness, and a lower risk of death (Safri, 2016), as well as indicators of psychological, subjective, and social well-being

(Long et al., 2020; Murphy, 2023). For instance, literature has identified outcomes associated with hope, which include a sense of competency in meeting goals, an ability to transcend the situation faced, and an understanding of overcoming the situation or having peace with it (Hasse et al., 1992). Hope has been significantly associated with better connectedness with others, and a better quality of life for people with mental illness and lower levels of hope and experiences of hopelessness were associated with lower mood and greater psychological distress (Hayes et al., 2017).

People who are hopeful can have a mindset of accomplishment; for instance, they can see barriers and hindrances as challenges to be overcome and create positive emotions and greater interest in activities (Oettingen & Gollwitzer, 2002). Higher levels of hope shape behaviour and increase persistence towards that which is hoped for, as well as having a better ability to cope with illness (e.g., Gum, 2017; Safri, 2016), and hope has been identified as promoting resilience (Goodman et al., 2017). Hope is also identified as a latent (underlying) factor which interacts with important psychological states to explain changes to quality of life. For instance, people with stroke who have higher hope experience less depression and perceived stress, which results in better quality of life (Fong et al., 2022). Review findings support this and have associated the cognitive and emotional aspects of hope with subjective well-being (Pleeging et al., 2021).

People that are hopeful are resilient, and hope is seen as an inner strength which enables persistence and resilience against adversity (Olsman, 2020). Hope appears so important to well-being that having false hope results in better outcomes for people than having no hope (Synder et al., 2002). For instance, in psychiatric research, hope has been associated with therapeuitc efficacy (Laranjeira & Querido, 2022), but a loss of hope has been assoicated with (Schrank et al., 2008). Further to this, hope appears to be particularly important at points of transition and change. At such points, hope can lead to more positive emotions and positively impact well-being (Ciarrochi et al., 2015).

Why being hopeful may not always be possible

Hope should be considered a good indicator of positive indices of health and is more influential on outcomes when the perception of control of a situation is high (Rand & Rogers, 2023). This view is complicated in chronic illness because what is hoped for may not be known with certainty (Soundy et al., 2016a). Further to this, perception of control can be restricted, which can impact on adjustment and experiences such as pain (Haythornthwaite et al., 1998). Hope may be prevented by the experience of suffering or the perceived inability to access a meaningful future (Soundy et al., 2014b). A meaningful future includes understanding how illness has impacted on meaningful relationships, roles, and

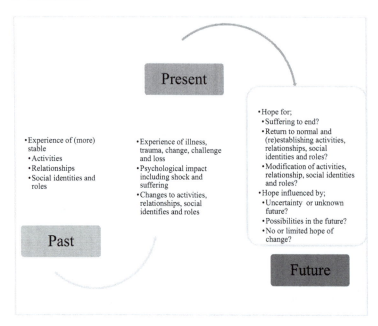

Figure 1.2 The importance of time alongside different levels of hope.

activities across time (Soundy et al., 2013). The expression of hope (Soundy et al., 2013) brings together aspects of time (past, present, and future) alongside the different levels of hope which act as the source of this expression (Soundy et al., 2014c). This includes what has been lost from the past and what the future could or may not be. Figure 1.2 considers how time may interact with the different levels of hope. The levels of hope illustrate the importance of reducing or removing suffering, once this has been achieved hope may more easily be identified in relationship to what is meaningful to the individual.

The most important hope is to stop suffering that is the likely cause of such experiences (Soundy et al., 2014b). Suffering is important to understand because it is regarded as the most important level of hope or what individuals will hope to stop as part of the illness. Suffering is identified as an embodied experience and defined as an unpleasant or even anguishing experience which severely affects a person at a psychophysical (internal and physical) and an existential level (how we decide to exist in the world and live life) (Bueno-Gómez, 2017). Suffering can be associated with distress from events that threaten the intactness of the person (Cassel, 2004), or is seen as a change in how the individual understands themselves in terms of losses or reconstruction of identities or roles (e.g., Charmaz, 1983). It is important to note that there is not a single way to suffer (Kleinman, 1997), and the sources of suffering are multiple and include social problems like social exclusion and internal and existential experiences like grief, helplessness, anguish, despair, nausea, fear, or physical pain (Bueno-Gómez, 2017). The experience of suffering can be all consuming, being able to hope, outside the desire for suffering to end may not be possible because the situation or circumstance, leaves no mental distance from it, or ability to get a moment of relief from it. Lynch (1965) defined hope as being able to see a future and a way out of a difficulty. A person who is suffering often will hope for it to stop. When it does not stop, the experience can become a trial and be considered a state which the individual is captive to, and this leads to an existence where the capacity to hope is prevented (Marcel, 1951). As such, it is important to acknowledge the ability for suffering to change over time as situations change (Nowotny, 1989). One important role of healthcare professionals is to understand if there is suffering or challenges faced by the individual before establishing goals and hopes.

Is a way out of suffering achievable in all circumstances?

It is possible that the circumstance surrounding suffering may provide an opportunity to create or receive something of value and/or to find meaning. Being able to find meaning is what authors (DuFault & Martoochio, 1985; Soundy et al., 2014a, 2014b; Wiles et al., 2008) refer to as a generalised hope. It is essential that when an individual considers hope it is for something that is meaningful (Stephenson, 1991). Hope is closely associated with meaning in life (Nekolaichuk et al., 1999) and protects against the experience of despair (Wiles et al., 2008). Rather than focusing on what was lost it may be more important to focus on how meaning in the present situation can be gained. Gibson (2017) suggests the ability to find meaning changes the individual's perception of suffering, from being a victim of suffering to becoming a survivor. Meaning (and therefore hope) for people with chronic illness can be found within an individual's social roles, perhaps as a father, their social identities, such as a worker like a teacher, or a club they belong to; further meaning is also found in social relationships with family and friends and in being able to engage in desired activities. Thus before, goals are made understanding what is meaningful for patients should be sought.

How is hope expressed when someone is suffering?

Being able to identify meaningful hopes and wishes may not be straight forward. Following the onset of chronic illness, the impact may be so great that surviving each day or each moment is the primary concern. Hope at such a point may be redefined and seen as the ability to keep going, not to be in despair, not to be, or feel, so broken. Depending on the context of an individual's situation and what is faced, seeing life as hopeless can be a result. The importance of hope at such a point is illustrated well by Frankl (2004) who identifies an existential vacuum which can result in death. Thus, suffering restricts and prevents certain hopes, if someone is suffering it seems perfectly normal to me that there may be no ability to identify a goal or to be motivated to achieve that goal. Suffering therefore may prevent what authors (DuFault & Martoochio, 1985; Soundy et al., 2014b; Wiles et al., 2008) call particularised hopes (those hopes which are specific and related to some level of recovery from a condition), which can often be the focus of rehabilitation.

One of the core goals of my work is to find an efficient way for healthcare professionals to identify if there is a challenge which is causing suffering or preventing hope. This is undertaken by getting the individual to identify their primary or greatest challenge faced in the present and then assessing how and if they can be hopeful and psychologically and emotionally adapt and respond to that challenge. Some definitions of hope suggest that if hope can be created it is indeed possible. For instance, Farren et al (1995) defined hope as "*inner power that facilitates the transcendence of the present situation and enables a reality-based expectation of a brighter tomorrow for self and/or others*". Further to this, Farran and McCann (1989) state that hope is based on the solution to problems presented and a way out of difficulty. Indeed, a hopeful state is associated with feelings of energy and being able to psychologically adapt (Stephenson, 1991). Other works provide examples of how hope can exist despite suffering. For instance, the work of Frankl (2004) illustrates that it is possible for individuals to find meaning in life despite suffering.

Hope is a subjective state (Farran & Popovich, 1990) which has a basis within personal experience (Owen, 1989). For instance, it is considered a feeling, emotion, or need (Tutton et al., 2009). Thus, to understand hope it would seem important to understand emotions. Both positive and negative emotions have been associated with hope. For instance, the experience of peace has been associated with hope, as has grief, if the objective ones hope for must end or be abandoned (Kylmä & Vehviläinen-Julkunen, 1997). Thus, feelings are linked to hope, and specific negative feelings as identified above (like despair) are considered the opposite of hope. The ability to understanding feelings and how they are associated with hope is required as part of creating a deeper understand of psychological adaptation.

Further to this, in order to find a way out of difficulty or challenge, an individual must be able to understand how people psychologically adapt and respond to present circumstances and how and if they can look forward to the future (Soundy, 2018). The ability to adapt is linked to the past and influenced by factors which affect hope (including, but not limited to supportive relationships, the provision of information, and past experiences), as well as being able to see different possibilities for the future. Thus adaptation requires a consideration of the hope for the future and the ability to accept in the present (Soundy et al., 2016a; 2016b). Hope and acceptance are two concepts which have been identified as intertwined and have been postulated to be powered by the same or similar processes (Lazarus, 1999). Farran et al. (1995) identifies one central component of hope is the acceptance and experience of trials as a part of being human. However, the ability to accept the present circumstances cannot be assumed, and how someone responds to a challenge, event, or trauma must be understood in terms of the ability to accept as well as the ability to look forward (Soundy et al., 2016b). For people with chronic illness, or for those facing very difficult circumstances, understanding the ability to have acceptance with a situation or being able to adapt and understand negative outcomes may not initially be possible. The following chapters of this book consider these central components of psychological adaptation and hope in more details.

Key points

- One core definition of hope has not been established. Rather hope is more often understood according to specific elements or factors. Most research has considered hope in terms of goals. This requires an individual to have agency (goal directed energy) and identify pathways (ways to achieve the goal).
- It is important to identify if individuals are not ready to identify a goal or able to see a way forward chronic illness. Within the definition of hope, uncertainty or threats may prevent the hope from occurring. Thus, being able to meet the demands of a threat or identify possible ways forward is important.
- During experiences of suffering, the broader elements of hope need to be considered through a process of understanding an individual's experience. Understanding suffering is important as this influences hope through the experience of emotions and psychological adaptation.
- Suffering will impact the ability to hope, so it must be addressed, and challenges faced by the individual identified before meaningful hopes can be identified.
- Hope should be considered alongside what an individual expresses as meaningful to them. This could include roles, social identities, activities, and relationship, and these aspects can often be a focus of hope for people with chronic illness.

Conclusion

Given the above introduction, I believe it is possible to understand why individuals who face suffering trauma or challenge may not be ready and motivated to identify goals, and it is possible to understand where this book is heading in terms of the need to understand more about the broader elements of hope. The following chapters further the focus and understanding of hope, how it is expressed and what factors influence it. The chapters then provide consideration of a tool currently used to enable hope-centred interactions.

2 Hope in chronic illness

Introduction

The subjective experience of time is viewed as a psychological concept that is constructed and reconstructed by people (Block, 1990). It is important to recognise that what is imagined in the past, present, or future is associated with an emotional reaction and a preference for specific action (Lennings, 1996). For instance, past negative perspectives and fatalistic views of the present have been associated with negative emotions such as anger, depression, or anxiety (Zimbardo & Boyd, 1999). Being able to switch between the past, present, and future flexibly represents a balanced time perspective (Zimbardo & Boyd, 1999), which is important to obtain optimal bio-psychosocial health (Zimbardo, 2002). However, individuals can become influenced to look at and focus on one perspective, which can become a dispositional characteristic and prevent healthy functioning (Soundy et al., 2013). It is essential that individuals avoid bias towards how time is regarded as this supports healthy functioning (Boniwell & Zimbardo, 2004). It has long been identified that how people perceive their future severs as a critical motivation for their thoughts and behaviours (Lewin, 1951). Having future-orientated coping strategies is essential to support the well-being of people who have chronic illness (Venning et al., 2008). The perception of the future is important because it acts as a motivating force for behaviour as well as influencing coping mechanisms like repression (Livneh, 2012). In chronic illness, several factors influence hope and the ability to look forward. This includes factors such as how and if the symptoms of the illness change, the severity levels of the illness, the illness prognosis and if it is deteriorating in nature, or the response the individual has to rehabilitation (Soundy et al., 2014c). It is important to understand what the future looks like, including if it is perceived as known or not about the challenge or situation, if the situation, challenge, or circumstances are deteriorating for the individual, and what can be identified as possible across different areas of life when considering the situation challenge or circumstances. Below different considerations of the future are explored in more detail to consider challenges and opportunities for looking forward and maintaining a psychologically healthy outlook.

DOI: 10.4324/9781003466161-2

Unknown or uncertain futures

The unknown or uncertain future may result from an experience of shock at diagnosis, an experience which has been described as the ground falling away or not wanting to believe what is happening (Leite et al., 2021). When the future is unknown, directions or pathways towards a desired goal are unknown (Wright, 1983). Higher levels of uncertainty created by a negative prognosis can reduce motivation to comply with treatment (Apóstolo et al., 2007). This experience can be surrounded by negative emotions such as grief, loss and despair created because of the uncertainty when looking forward (Lohne & Severinsson, 2004). The unpredictable nature of an illness can mean experiences can oscillate between hope and despair (Laskiwski & Morse, 1993). For instance, in a study by Sällfors et al. (2002) one child with chronic illness stated:

> "You get so disappointed, because suddenly you're better . . . and then your worse again. All the time your hoping you will get better". Another child said "It was dreadful . . . because I thought I'd die then . . . I said to Mum . . . I can't cope. . . . Will it be like this for a whole week? I didn't know what to do".

Time points in the course of a chronic illness can increase uncertainty of the future, this includes when waiting for diagnosis, or following diagnosis an unknown future may be associated with the illness or disease because of its unpredictable nature (Sällfors et al., 2002). Specific sources of uncertainty have been identified by (Hinton & Kirk, 2017); this can include (a) diagnostic uncertainty, which is created because of difficulty in diagnosing the illness and complicated by different healthcare professionals required for the diagnosis and/or conflicting opinions about the diagnosis; (b) uncertainty caused by how unknown or unpredictable symptoms makes planning and preparation for daily activities difficult; (c) uncertainty causes by interactions especially if the illness is not believed or disputed, this could occur more during periods of remission; and (d) future uncertainty created by a lack of an ability to identify a prognosis and plan for the future. Another study relates the experiences of multiple sclerosis to existential uncertainty, where the body, sense of self and life are constantly threatened (Mazanderani et al., 2017).

Despite the above, uncertainty is not always considered bad or associated with negative feelings; some people seek out uncertainty-inducing activities like watching a sport and not knowing the outcome (Anderson et al., 2019). In chronic illness, the seeking out of uncertainty, unknown, and potentially detrimental situations was observed in a study by Alawafi et al. (2022). One patient identified what could be termed an adventure narrative, where new and novel experiences were sought and presented as an adventure, even when negative experiences occur like falling over or becoming injured was part of the story.

It is important for healthcare professionals to recognise the impact of uncertainty, especially during a downward trajectory of an illness or acute phase of illness where uncertainty has a greater impact on people (Mishel, 1990). In a temporal sequence, it would seem most likely that the experience of uncertainty precedes the experience of possibility or the ability to identify different ways to look forward and identify what may be possible. Uncertainty may be associated with specific emotions, particularly the emotion of fear. It is important to recognise that fear is a very strong emotion and fear of the unknown is the strongest kind of fear, and this can represent a basic component of anxiety (Carleton, 2016). Thus, being able to identify and acknowledge points of uncertainty for a patient is highly valuable because these points are more likely associated with worry or fears or other negative emotions, cognitions, and behaviours.

Negative, limited, or unwanted futures

Often at the beginning of an event, trauma or illness individuals can hold on to a hope of being restored. Being restored means using the past as a reference point to get back to and can represent the biggest hopes for patients, restoration can relate to past social identities or activities or be represented by critical tasks such as walking (Soundy et al., 2023). The idea of restoration often represents what life was like before the illness or what was considered normal. Being restored is a natural hope, this hope could be expressed in the absence of knowledge and understanding as well as with the promise of novel treatment (Leite et al., 2021). This expression may include denying present realities, hoping instead for an illness that does not progress or alternative diagnosis (Pinto et al., 2023). The perception of a negative future may be instigated by experiences of a lack of continued improvement during rehabilitation, failure to achieve goals set or slowing improvement (Soundy et al., 2014c). The experience of progressive disease such as motor neurone disease can impact an individual significantly and negatively at the point of diagnosis. At such a point in time, the future can be seen as having no direction or bleak but also as identifying future lives being cut off (Ziebland & Renata, 2012). One study on people with multiple sclerosis identified the most feared symptom as loss of mobility; one participant identified this as being chased by a monster called wheelchair bound (Mazanderani et al., 2019). Such experiences, like the onset of an illness, could create fear, frustration, perceptions of powerlessness, and continued suffering. Continued suffering is particularly important, and physical or psychological suffering could be so great that an individual hopes to die (Pinto et al., 2023). Where a disease is very aggressive, risks of seeking out medication can become a solution, even where the solution has its own risks to health (Mazanderani et al., 2017). Suffering can make people feel that life is not worth living, and this is often within the context of having previously attempted many treatment options (Sällfors et al., 2002). If time in the future is limited, it can reduce hope (de Graaf, 2016), and hope can be lost at moments where it is identified that nothing further can be done to change the situation (Leite et al., 2021). Feelings of hopelessness can suggest that the future is constricted and foreshortened and this often means goals and future plans are disregarded (Livneh, 2013). Further to this, suffering and thinking about dying can prevent individuals from using the resource of hope, create fear, increase the experience of pain, and ultimately be associated with the cause of death (Pinto et al., 2023).

Possible futures

Whilst a lack of hope can exist before an inevitable outcome, this may not mean the person cannot rise above the circumstance (Marcel, 1951). There may be different conditions needed for this. For instance, Penz and Duggleby (2011) within their research define hope as "*a positive or optimistic state of being, involving a perseverant and realistic understanding of future possibilities*" (p. 286). Understanding what is perceived possible and the different avenues of possibility across many meaningful aspects of life is essential when promoting hope. Hope may only begin or continue from a point of view that individuals can look forward and desire a future with meaningful activities, identities, or roles (Mairami et al., 2020; Bright et al., 2019). To enable a view of looking for different possibilities, it is likely that some form of acknowledgement is needed. This includes an acknowledgement of (a) what has happened in the present situation and (b) that, to some extent, the ability to control a situation may be limited (Soundy & Condon, 2015). When considering hope and possibility, the degrees and depth of hope vary from global hopes like peace, to hope for suffering to end, to hope of something more mundane like a certain cake left in a cake shop. More depth is involved in the hope to find meaning in illness, but being able to do this promotes the experience of enjoyment and pleasure (Stempsey, 2015). Creating a possible future will involve understanding the meaning identified by the individual with chronic illness, and the individual may require time and support before they can identify this.

Hoping despite the future

People do not need to give up all hope. As well as having a realistic understanding of future possibilities, possible futures may only be possible by not accepting that life is over. According to Marcel (1951), hope is a non-acceptance of being doomed by fate. Alternatively, Pruyser (1963) identifies, people can respond to a prognosis where no cure is possible by acknowledging this prognosis, yet still hoping, where they demonstrate acceptance and understanding of their future reality but still hope. A good example of this within my own clinical work was when an individual who had suffered a stroke came to the community rehabilitation centre where I was running classes and wanted to join. He stated that the physiotherapists he worked with said there was no point in continuing rehabilitation because it would not make him any better. I agreed to support him on the basis that attending the classes regardless of improvement would benefit his physical and mental health, that the community classes represented a positive environment, that he would have access to positive peer role models, have an opportunity to meet and be supported by students regardless of the outcome, and also that a lack of hope can mean there is no meaning or purpose, and this can create a vicious cycle of despair (Soundy et al., 2013). Thus, hope can be found across the different levels of hope that exist (Soundy et al., 2014c).

It may be that when uncertainty is greatest, the hopes an individual has must be more general before they can be more specific. Workovers during the lockdowns in the UK were valuable for considering hope, for instance, during the first research study to use to support physiotherapy students. Soundy et al. (2021a) were able to illustrate how uncertainty leaves room for more general ways of looking forward only, illustrating that specific hopes, desires, or expectations were removed to leave a view of hope created as (a) the situation will get better whilst acknowledging how this will happen is not known, (b) hope that the situation would pass and normality would return, and (c) a general hope that there will be a better future or a time in the future where things would be better.

Hope from a more certain future

Hope for the future can be expressed by having a good outcome from rehabilitation or more concrete than this of having a miracle cure (Soundy et al., 2014a). Depending on the illness or condition, hope can be gained through information such as doctors identifying that a tumour is reducing in size (Leite et al., 2021). A more certain future can be established at such times, and it may also be that patients understand the impact of the condition and the importance of modifying how and if restoration of activities, relationships, and identities can be established. Creating a more certain future through experience, rehabilitation, and understanding of how others have adapted provides hope and a better ability to adapt to the present circumstances.

Key points

- Uncertainty of the future can precede and prevent the identification of possibilities for the future, blinding people to hope. Uncertainty appears worse during an acute phase or illness or when an illness has no or a negative prognosis, which impacts the ability to hope.

- Uncertainty can create negative emotions, which means individuals can easily oscillate between hope and despair. However, experiences of uncertainty can be considered different, and there are examples of people with chronic illness seeking out uncertainty.
- Understanding worries, fears, and other negative emotions is essential to help relieve and reconsider hope for the future.
- Multiple and different future possibilities need to be identified to create a meaningful future. Identifying and promoting meaningful activities, roles, and relationships are essential to this.
- Part of being hopeful may involve a non-acceptance of being doomed by a probably outcome. Allowing this expression may be essential at times of greatest threat or uncertainty.

Conclusion

The future of people with chronic illness can be significantly impacted by the uncertainty of illness. However, uncertainty may not always be viewed as a negative experience. Being able to identify different meaningful hopes to create different and varied futures is important to promote hope. However, allowing the expression of non-acceptances may be equally important when considering interactions that relate towards the future.

3 Strategies that enhance possible, restored, and certain futures

Introduction

Research on hope often reveals significant factors, which influence the experience of hope within chronic illness. This chapter provides the first considerations of factors that influence hope (Soundy et al., 2014c). From the research in Chapter 2, it has been established that a sense of meaning and purpose may stem from the different levels of hope, including reducing suffering and finding meaning from relationships, roles, and social identities, as well as activities. Chapter 3 provides an identification of how and why the future may seem difficult to consider. This chapter furthers this past by identifying practical ways to enable hope for people with chronic illness. Several factors are identified and explored as follows: (a) creating meaning for people; (b) identifying aims and goals; (c) drawing on one's own positive personal characteristic; and finally, (d) creating possible futures.

Creating meaning for people

Past losses around roles, perception of control around aspects of life or symptoms of illness, health, income, support, and interest from others can decrease hope (Soundy et al., 2014c; Olsman, 2021). To enhance hope, it is important that different areas of life are considered, and individuals identify what is personally meaningful to themselves (Herth, 1995). What is meaningful can be a goal, a solution to a problem, relief from suffering, an activity, or relationship (Dufault & Martocchi, 1985). Meaning is especially valuable if the illness becomes palliative experiences that can be accessed within the present become more important (Ersek, 1992; Miller, 1991, 2007). This may include listening to music, reading books, having food, or enjoying experiences outside. Long et al. (2020) identified a significant positive association between hope with physical activity, mastery volunteering, and having a sense of purpose in life. Meaningful relationships are just as important to this (Herth, 1990). Being able to identify meaningful activities is important to ensure motivation for activities selected. Finding meaningful activities that

DOI: 10.4324/9781003466161-3

are enjoyed will positively influence their motivation. This is supported by past literature on motivation (Wigfield & Eccles, 2000).

Meaning and hope can also be enhanced by complying with rehabilitation, and this can create a greater perception of personal control and provide access to improvements or turning points is something referred to by Soundy et al. (2013) as "active hope". This supported by other literature which has found that people who are more conscientious (a characteristic that is associated with people who have a high sense of self-control, who are purposeful in their action and self-disciplined) can adjust to a chronic illness more effectively (Helgeson & Zajdel, 2017). At points during rehabilitation, hope could be enhanced further, including achieving milestones within rehabilitation or from meaningful achievements like gaining a role or mastering an activity (Soundy et al., 2014c). Further to this, successful experiences can lead to the creation of further plans and goals (Alawafi et al., 2022).

Identifying aims or goals

Meaningful and tailored goals that can adapt and change to circumstances and change to bring the timeframe closer to enable goal attainment enhance hope (Soundy et al., 2014c). Progress towards goals creates positive emotions, whereas a lack of progress can lead to negative emotions (Ciarrochi et al., 2015). This can be helped by identifying short-term aims that are more focused on the present. In addition to this as well as the ability to devise and revise goals (Herth, 1995; Simpson, 2004). To enable goals individuals should be supported with specific aims that are attainable (Herth, 1990; 1993) and be supported to devise and revise goals (Herth, 1995; Simpson, 2004). Interventions that use Synder's hope theory identify three main elements when considering goals (Weis & Speridkos, 2011), including (a) the need to identify meaningful goals, if needed broken into accomplishable parts; (b) the identification of what hope theory is, as well as identifying the important components of pathway and agency thinking; and (c) finally, narratives that can be used to target agency thinking, meaning that accessible stories of others are able to aid the establishment of goals. Successful goal attainment enables individuals to implement goals by themselves and understand how to achieve them (Ciarrochi et al., 2015).

Identifying oneself or characteristics

Being able to relate to one's personality attributes like determination and persistence can be valuable to hope (Soundy et al., 2014c). Other studies have identified similar attributes which enable hope including resilience, patience, and courage (Schrank et al., 2008). Such positive characteristics enable individuals to act autonomously (Pinto et al., 2023). This is supported by other research for instance value of characteristics such as serenity, courage, or determination were identified by Herth (1995) or being "bloody minded", determined to prove others wrong or motivated not to let others down was identified by Alawafi et al.

(2022). These traits are likely part of an individual's positive character (Ols-man, 2021) or attitude (Penz & Duggleby, 2011). Such characteristics may also represent or be part of a philosophy of life that conveys a sense of optimism, personal growth through difficulties, and meaning gained from experiences. It may be something the individual relates to part of themselves (Soundy et al., 2012), and it may provide a greater sense of self to the individual, which acts to protect against future psychological difficulties (Venning et al., 2008). Finally, such characteristics demonstrate a future-looking orientation or attitude, which has been considered a personality trait (Gorman & Wessman, 1977). In sum-mary, understanding an individual's character may be especially important for hope. Specific questions during rehabilitation about positive attributes of the individual's character that existed before the chronic illness may benefit the present circumstances and enable a future-orientated outlook.

Establishing possible futures

There are different ways of creating possible futures. The following five ways are considered:

(a) Ensuring that an individual can see different and varied opportunities that are possible. The focus and consideration given to different and varied hopes for the future can be important, especially where something that is hoped is not possible to obtain. A study by Kylmä and Vehviläinen-Julkunen (1997) suggests that it is important to identify or picture differ-ent possibilities acknowledging the opportunity and limitations of those possibilities at the same time. It may represent a search for information on research which is already known to put a jigsaw together about what is known, and this stance requires an active and investigative role for the individual with chronic illness (Lacerda et al., 2019). It can also reflect doing activities in different ways. For instance, where a grandparent can-not lift their grandchildren, they may be able to undertake an alternative activity with them (Kralik et al., 2004). Finally, it may require a continual adjustment of the concept of self, which requires discarding old activities and re-discovering new activities (Subramanian et al., 2024).

(b) Hope can be enabled by not looking to far forward at hopes that may not be possible, and it may be that looking forward to the next one day or getting through the next hour is needed, especially in very challenging situations (Soundy et al., 2014c). Being able to focus on current issues can provide an opportunity for individuals to consider the future (Livneh, 2013). Not looking too far in the future may be enhanced by a process of reconciliation with what is currently possible, as this will help indi-viduals find new meaning (Pinto et al., 2023) but also by refocusing on "small wins" or small joys in the present (Herth, 1995). This can help an individual embrace the different situations and challenges that the illness could bring because of its unknown or changing nature (Soundy et al., 2012). When considering activities, it is important that the enjoyment of the activity be established. For instance, feelings of fatigue are rarely observed when an individual is interested in the task they are performing; enjoyment of activities is associated with more energy and elation and can be sustained for longer (Hockey, 2011).

(c) Using imagination as a way forward and what life could be like. This could mean thinking about the situation differently and being able to identify benefits or growth that has results (Soundy & Condon, 2015). Part of this process requires creativity around the different ways out of a challenge or difficulty (Simpson, 2004), and it could also include visualising one's self in the future (Livneh, 2013; Smith, 2008) and imaging different possible futures (Ref_29_FILE240440003BM1De Graaf, 2016). It could include contrasting what life would be like if changes are made versus if they are not made (Hardcastle et al., 2015). Imagination may play a role in identifying a future hope that is possible, and this goes beyond calculating the probability of something happening (Stempsey, 2015). However, at times, it may only be possible when concerns are bracketed and information on risk reinterpreted to avoid the thoughts of futures which are more negative (Brown & de Graaf, 2013).

(d) Making a choice to live in a way that defies the limitations that is presented by an illness. Some patients would create a personal challenge to defy the illness. This could include by maintaining their past social identities or creating specific challenges to overcome (Soundy et al., 2012). An example of this included finding ways to physically overcome obstacles like climbing the stairs using their hands. This example identifies the importance of individuals finding boundaries in what is possible through attempting activities (Kralik et al., 2004). This can represent an acknowledgement of what had happened but also illustrated a non-acceptance of the impact and restrictions that may be identified by others including healthcare professionals. A good example of non-acceptance was generated in a study considering people with multiple sclerosis (Synder et al., 2014). The study focuses on people who were denied access to therapy and so travelled abroad to receive it. The hope of stopping the progressive nature of the MS was identified as the dominant emotion which aided the decision. The decision was guided by their own research, peers, and the assessment of credentials of physicians that would provide the treatment. Other choices identified by past research (Haahr et al., 2011) include making the most of a situation or living according to a routine without the need for help, for as long as that is possible.

(e) Another way to enable possibility was considered being able to reconciling and reconsidering hopes to find new avenues (Penz & Duggleby, 2011). This may also be known or identified as value changes or benefit finding. People who can identify benefits and value experiences following adversity tend to demonstrate better adjustment (McAdams et al., 2001).

Often, this includes the idea that something can be gained from the experience, and this may include identifying problems with care that you want to be a part of changing or seeing life as an adventure despite negative experiences occurring (Alawafi et al., 2022). Alternatively, this could also include redefining or reviewing hopes, and this is important when specific hopes were not obtained (Herth, 1995) and this helps individuals reconsider hope and find new avenues for hope (Penz & Duggleby, 2011). Ersek (1992) identified that redefining hopes within rationale thought processes which also include reflecting on reality and reviewing past successes is important for psychological adaptation. Work has reported that being able to identify achievements, advocating for the disease and giving back to others are associated with feelings of optimism for people (Gardenhire et al., 2019). The association between benefit finding and adjustment to disease has support; however, it does not imply that this will reduce psychological distress (Helgeson & Zajdel, 2017). Healthcare professionals may need to help patients adapt or redirect hopes to allow this process to occur (Soundy et al., 2014c).

(f) Having hope despite the outcome. Authors have highlighted that maintaining positivity has been identified as a factor that influences hope (Reynolds & Prior, 2003). Being able to keep a positive attitude or view is considered important (Wiles et al., 2008) despite obstacles, disappointments, and challenges (Penz & Duggleby, 2011). Being able to identify areas of hopelessness and not letting those areas pollute other areas of possibility are important to this (Lynch, 1965). This may be enhanced by considering other positive-related situations and demonstrates potential opportunities for hope from others (Mishel, 1990). To maintain positive thinking at times may require not talking about the illness or problem (Pinto et al., 2023) or may require individuals to leave the door open to hope (Soundy et al., 2014c).

The idea of being positive has been referred to as the illusion belief of a generally positive outcome (Mishel, 1990). It is important to recognise that as an initial response to change, challenge, or loss false hope can be associated with better health outcomes than no hope (Synder et al., 2002), and having some hope is needed to be able to continue living. One parent in a study by Conway et al. (2017) speaking of their personal experience of having a child who had cancer said, *"Hope is knowing that even in the midst of the absolute worst that everything will still be okay"*. Other studies have reported individuals who are able to be hopeful are less affected by the disease (Bright et al., 2019) and by personal limitation or severity as it has on their life role (Cross & Schnider, 2010).

Finally, healthcare professionals should not forget the importance of faith for people as it can be a source of hope despite outcomes. According to Marcel, ultimate hope is rooted in religious belief (Marcel, 1951), and many spiritual belief systems provide peace in the hope of life after death (Parker-Oliver, 2002). In research, it has been identified that hope is facilitated by spiritual beliefs and practices (Herth, 1995; Kylmä et al., 1996). As identified within the definition of hope, the concept of faith and belief in God provides access to hope, especially in suffering where faith can act as a strong motivator to endure suffering, enhance agency, and encourage individuals to achieve goals (Nell & Rothmann, 2018). Religious text can provide a context of this; for instance, in Saint Paul's letter to the Philippians, he identifies an internal strategy to enable hope "*one thing I do: Forgetting what is behind and straining towards what is ahead*" (Chapter 3, verse 13). The context of this quote is following identifying participation in sufferings (3:10). Faith can help people even to the point of death (Conway et al., 2017) as faith gives hope meaning (Herth, 1995; Kylmä et al., 1996).

Key points

Being able to harness hope will be aided by the following factors:

- Being able to identify meaningful goals that, if needed, can be adjusted and adapted is important to the creation of hope.
- Goal setting is important to creating hope including breaking down goals to accomplishable parts, consider agency and pathways and narratives of others to help identify pathways, and enable agency.
- Individuals may have previously identified with positive characteristics such as determination, courage, or resilience. It may be possible to consider this characteristic pre-event or illness to use them to inform a future response.
- Specific internal or psychological strategies can be extremely valuable, including identifying different and varied hopes and opportunities, not looking too far ahead if those hopes are not immediately accessible, using imagination to see different possible futures, choosing to live in a way that defies situations, reconciling, reframing, or benefit finding, and having hope despite the outcome.
- When individuals are not motivated to change behaviour, it may be that exploration of values are undertaken and that those aspects that are most important are linked to rehabilitation and change. This is an aspect supported by other well-respected research like motivational interviewing (Miller & Rollnick, 2013)
- Hope should be considered a something that can exist despite specific outcomes. Hope will can often depend on the viewpoint and experiences of the individual and may be supported by an individual's faith in God.

Conclusion

It is essential that practical strategies that enable hope are considered by healthcare professionals and patients or people who are facing challenges. Being able to use and access such strategies could make the difference between being able to create positive change and not.

4   Sources of support
and encouragement

Introduction

Social support and relationships (professional and persona) are valuable to hope. Some authors have identified hope as having a relational component (Hammer et al., 2009). In relationships where love is received and given people can be encouraged, feel more hopeful and be affirmed by each other. This can provide individuals with a sense of support and worth. People who receive positive support (perceived as being cared for and encouraged) are more hopeful (Kim et al., 2006). When people are in need, others around them can be carriers of hope (Sælør et al., 2014). In addition to this, positive relationships have been associated with establishing trust and finding meaning, purpose, and confidence (Schrank et al., 2009). Literature has consistently recognised the importance of relationships and interactions as factors, which can positively or negatively influence hope.

Despite the importance of relationships to hope, many healthcare professionals do not know how to instil hope to patients (Qama et al., 2022), and it is an activity which healthcare professionals need to work at and be an active participant in (Penz & Duggleby, 2011). Hope is often considered in the context of goal setting within a therapeutic conversation but limited by an assumption around the restoration of function as a desired future (Bright et al., 2024). This chapter will provide further understanding of the value of relationships and interactions on hope and identify the role social support plays in enhancing hope. The chapter will finish by focusing on the importance of therapeutic interactions with healthcare professionals.

Relationships and connection with others

Several studies acknowledged the importance of meaningful relationships and being connected with others (e.g., Ersek, 1992; Herth, 1990, 1995;

DOI: 10.4324/9781003466161-4

Kylmä et al., 1996; Olsman, 2021). Relationships help limit isolation (Ersek, 2006) and allow the sharing of experiences (Kylmä et al., 1996), provide the experience of closeness from an important (Long et al., 2021), and enable someone to feel part of something or feel needed. Interactions can increase hope, and this includes being near others who radiate hope or just having others present in moments (Herth, 1990). The ability to share experiences is important (Kylmä & Vehviläinen-Julkunen, 1997). One particularly useful part of interactions is the ability to share and consider possibilities with others (Simpson, 2004). Individuals benefit from positive stories from others (Olsman, 2021).

The provision of support is a central factor which facilitates hope, and this can be seen in several ways according to Soundy et al. (2014c). This includes peer support, as it provides motivation and encouragement, understanding of others journey has been identified as meaningful as it can be deeper than other relationships. It also provides access to models of behaviour, thoughts, and action, which can encourage hope. It can be from family or from those that listen, encourage, and provide information. Support from peers is valuable during a time of turmoil (Sällfors et al., 2002). Hope from relationships is often generated from being encouraged or supported in times of need (Leite et al., 2021). The presence of another person who provides tolerance, understanding, and unconditional acceptance can increase hope (Miller, 2007). However, it should be noted that individuals can be very aware of the importance of not becoming a burden to others (Pinto et al., 2023).

Two major factors which remove hope include when someone feels unsupported or when they feel isolated. The nature of being unsupported is identified by Soundy et al. (2014c) as the ability to share and/or the ability to be heard by someone else; this may be as simple as a healthcare professional or significant other not having sufficient time to listen or lacking empathy. Being unsupported may also represent partners that leave the patient because of the illness and what it means. The experience of isolation or abandonment may be emotional or physical loss of others, and emotional withdrawal has been considered worse than physical withdrawal (Herth, 1990).

Responses to hope from healthcare professionals

Healthcare professionals are often not identified as a source of hope but often can remove hope (Robichaud & Simpson, 2013). In particular circumstances, patients may avoid or dismiss the value of a healthcare professional because they removed hope (Soundy et al., 2012). Alternatively, particular healthcare professionals may be sought because of how they instil hope or may be identified because of the opportunity they can provide. For instance, if they provide a novel treatment and have a good reputation and experience, this can create hope (Mazanderani et al., 2017). The provision of information during chronic illness is never more important than when patient goals and priorities of the future do not align with the professional's view (Hill et al., 2023). Reder and Serwint (2009) identify that healthcare professionals can view the prognosis of a chronic illness in tension against the need to accept the reality of the illness, whereas parents of the severely ill children saw the concepts as co-existing. Some healthcare professionals may perceive a need or pressure to inform or correct understanding. However, the manner of the message when conveying limited or no hope to patients requires consideration, and hope can be removed through a lack of empathy or limited time to listen and understand losses experienced (Soundy et al., 2014c). One patient in the study by Alawafi et al. (2021) noted the danger of healthcare professionals introducing false despair. Being able to manage this conflict is essential for any clinician.

Bright et al. (2024) identify how healthcare professionals limit conversations about the future. This occurs through pragmatic needs within the hospital setting and getting people with chronic illness to discharge rather than looking beyond discharge. Further to this, it was noted that only a few conversations appeared to attend to patients' meaningful activities or roles, social identity, or emotions. Rather, healthcare professionals frequently focused on assumed desires and wants around past functioning and chose not to consider broader goals that may have meaning to the patient or consider more distant or unknown futures. In addition to this, healthcare professionals may prefer certain responses from patients within rehabilitation. Healthcare professionals may encourage outcomes which are considered in their view "realistic" and that embrace the future whilst acknowledging the present circumstances and discourage outcomes that demonstrate a "false hope", no hope, or a passive hope (Soundy et al., 2013). One problem with focusing on realistic hopes is that healthcare professionals do not give support to broader hopes, which in turn limits the ability to establish hope for the future (Bright et al., 2019). Inevitably the danger is that the management of hope and conversations about future are limited and experienced in a negative way by people with chronic illness (Soundy et al., 2012).

Hope has a central role in well-being; to remove it is like removing something the individual should live with much like the food we eat. Indeed, physical limitations and impact or illness severity may not change an individual's sense of hope because it is considered constant. However, having a sole focus on limitations and impairments can create a loss of hope (Cross & Schneider, 2010). In contrast, people who have suffered a stroke and who are facing deterioration overtime have been shown to identify goals and have greater levels of hope and energy than people with stroke who did not identify goals and did not have current experiences of deterioration (Soundy et al., 2023).

The promotion of hope

There are specific ways of engaging with patients to enable hope. For instance, hope is enhanced by the process of establishing rapport, which includes the provision of care, support, attention, and listening (Conway et al., 2017; Herth, 1995; Penz & Duggleby, 2011; Soundy et al., 2014c). These are considered essential aspects of emotional support which promote hope (Moss et al., 2021). Hope is decreased with non-caring responses (Herth, 1990). This may be complicated by healthcare professionals not understanding the role they have in having conversations regarding the future, especially where illness prognosis is poor (Momen et al., 2012). Within interactions, specific aspects of communication need to be considered. This includes feeling accepted and acknowledged (Herth, 1990; Kylmä et al., 1996), having the patient's sense of worth affirmed (Olsman, 2021), and enabling the patient to feel honoured (Herth, 1990; Kylmä et al., 1996). Hope can be reduced during periods of isolation (Long et al., 2021), and patients can experience fear of being abandoned or being institutionalised, which also decreases hope (Pinto et al., 2023). The experience of hope can also be lost through being told how to feel, for example, in the wrong circumstances being told *"you should feel lucky to be alive"*. Such responses can ignore the emotional impact of the experience and illustrate an unwillingness to understand the experience (Moss et al., 2021). Developing hope is important as it is associated with trust in a relationship (Brown, 2011), and it is a protective state for well-being (Rosenberg et al., 2021).

Several articles identified several important strategies during communication that would enhance hope. This included (a) promoting diverse, complex, and flexible hopes (Rosenbergy et al., 2021) and avoiding no hope (Synder et al., 2002); identifying and considering other possibilities; and considering hopes other than a cure (Rosenberg et al., 2021; Penz & Duggleby, 2011; Simpson, 2004). (b) The correction of "unrealistic hopes" as perceived by healthcare professionals can reduce hope (Rosenberg et al., 2021). It is essential to remember that hopes are not called or described as false unless an alternative course of action is considered by a professional (Lazarus, 1999). For an individual's health and well-being, false hope can be better than no hope (Synder et al., 2002). Being aware of this important aspect of hope will help to promote acceptance (Rosenberg et al., 2021). Further to this, healthcare professionals should be aware that patients can present an optimism bias during communication and be more confident in positive outcomes (Penz & Duggleby, 2011), (c) using light-heartedness or humour has been shown to enhance hope (Herth, 1995; Pinto et al., 2023; Soundy et al., 2014c), (d) being open in communication is important for patients and allows hope to be developed (Esek, 2006; Temple, 2017), (e) identifying treatments, medicine, or procedures that help is valuable for hope (Brown, 2011; Pinto et al., 2023; Temple, 2017) and provides a sense of security and certainty in situations that are often surrounded by uncertainty (Venning et al., 2008). Finally, (f) healthcare professionals should be attentive to metaphoric language used by patient as metaphors are consistently used to describe emotional experiences and can be explored within therapeutic conversations (Ziebland & Kokanovic, 2012).

Key points

Healthcare professionals should be aware of the following factors that relate to creating supportive interactions:

- Taking the time to listen and explore patients' responses to the challenges faced will help created a trusted partnership so people feel supported and not isolated.
- Being aware of a "medical voice" which labels responses in particular ways and limits experiences or stories as "unrealistic" may not be at all helpful.
- Conversations about hope can often be limited to a setting and focus on getting to discharge rather than beyond that time point. However, more focus on meaningful activities and relationships that link with an individual's wishes are important to consider.
- Understanding strategies that enhance hope is essential, including the need to promote diverse, flexible, and complex hopes, not correct what may initially be identified as false hopes unless another vision for hope is established, using humour or light-heartedness (further training is essential on this), being aware of and conveying possible treatment options, and being attentive to exploring language, especially the use of metaphors by patients.

Conclusion

It is essential that healthcare professionals recognise the importance of support for patients and how and why this can help or hinder how hopeful a patient feels. This chapter provides specific examples of this and should be considered and reflected upon to enable hope-centred interactions.

5 Understanding chronic illness through the expression of narratives

Introduction

Stephenson (1991) identified that hope had an orientation towards the future as positive but grounded in the present and associated with the past and something which has an element of anticipation. Life stories reveal how an individual expresses their own experiences in a unifying way from the past, to the present and future (Dunlop, 2022). One of the primary ways patients with chronic illness will share experiences of hope and time is using stories. Stories are used to illustrate how life is experienced and expressed, and they are easily shared, related to, and understood by people. Stories are often developed within particular settings, cultures, or groups. Gergen and Gergen (1997) identified that if an individual's actions are to be understood, then some form of temporal embedding is needed and events (such as illness, change, and the introduction of uncertainty) need to be understood by preceding and subsequent events. When individuals with chronic illness look forward, this can reflect different views of how their past is considered, and these different views of illness experiences can be captured by the master plots of chronic illness. Master plots are the most common and recognisable plots of stories or narratives (both terms in this chapter are used interchangeably) that express the experience of illness (Soundy et al., 2013). Importantly, these common plots convey hope and the time differently. Master plots consider the past, present, and future differently and illustrate some form of hope and psychological adaptation. In addition to this, they indicate how they want their story to be understood and provide a sense of meaning (Elliott, 2005).

The sharing of and listening to stories help create psychological movement for patients and promote psychological adjustment. Being able to access other stories can illustrate a lived example of different psychologically adaptive responses (Soundy, 2018). Within the narrative, there is often an end point which is linked to what has been identified as meaningful to the patient, and what is considered within the telling will make the end point or goal state either more or less probable. Before considering how to develop hope-centred interactions in the upcoming chapters, it is worth acknowledging how you

DOI: 10.4324/9781003466161-5

may hear hope when a patient or another person is speaking with you. Recognising the most common master plots is one way to do this, and each master plots contains different end points for people with chronic illness. Understanding the broad types of narrative is important because it is likely a primary way in which healthcare professionals will come to interact and guide hope, knowingly or unknowingly. This is important because certain stories can be limited, written off, silenced, and confronted with change (e.g., Soundy et al., 2010), whilst other stories are more acceptable following training (Alawafi et al., 2023). Below I provide a grouping of the most common types of plots associated with illness, and this has been summarised in Table 5.1.

Narratives that highlight a negative outcome, a downfall, or a limited future

Some master plots focus on what is lost from the past or how life has been impacted and changed (e.g., a tragic, regressive, chaos, or sad narrative). The end point of these master plots identifies what is not possible anymore. A regressive narrative can be affected by the lack of perceived control (Gergen & Gergen, 1997) and lacks a sense of investment in the future that comes from the promise of a valued future (Dunlop, 2022). These narratives may represent what McAdams et al. (2001) call a contamination sequence, which demonstrates how a positive life scene moves towards a bad, spoiled, or contaminated scene undermined by an event like a disruption or illness. One master plot that represents the most challenged outlook is called the chaos narrative, and this often lacks a plot as the teller is not able to look forward because of the loss and change experienced. This master plots identified no hope in the future or life worth living is termed the chaos narrative. Following clinical training, healthcare professionals appear less empathetic to this narrative and can associate it with a poor attitude toward rehabilitation (Soundy et al., 2010). These narratives need to be heard and supported accepting time needed to help them change may be significant.

Narratives that observe or review the events that have occurred

Two master plots provide an illustration of viewing events differently and reviewing events. These include the comic narrative and detached narrative, respectively. The value of comedy can be found in its ability to bring light-heartedness or fun to recovery as well as distance from living with a chronic illness (Declercq et al., 2024). The comic narrative considers looking at the present circumstances, past, or future differently, which may provide relief or some distance from the experience of illness, and it can allow other possibilities to be acknowledged and related to. Other stories focus on the journey, observing it as detached from emotions (termed a detached narrative). The goal state (or end point) of the narrative is identified by describing what happened, and the process of telling provides an opportunity to reframe the view of it. Such stories may have value as they are directly associated with internal strategies that enable hope identified in the past chapter.

Narratives that focus on a better future

Some narrative master plots identify the goal or end point is some form of restoration or redemptive state. These types of narratives have been referred to as progressive narratives. They highlight positive movement and highlight action undertaken. The restitution narrative is one of the most common master plots. People may express this master plot when there is a hope that the past will be restored completely, often this is through medicine or rehabilitation and can be seen as a concrete or certain hope for the future. A quote from a participant in a study by Toye and Barker (2012) highlights this: "*I plan to go back to everything . . . there is nothing that I will not do . . . I can't see any reason for stopping doing anything. I might have to do it differently, but, I can't see any reason . . . I go to the gym, I go swimming, I do everything that somebody that doesn't have a bad back does*" (p. 879). One problem with this narrative is if what is hoped for is not considered possible by others. Following training, healthcare students can identify the problems with the narrative as being "unrealistic" and "not accepted" (Soundy et al., 2010). Thus, this narrative may be one that healthcare professionals seek to change and modify. Using the above quote, it may be possible to see the flexibility presented by the individual in this case – that what is wanted could be done differently – but the danger of challenging the narrative without an alternative is that the future may appear to be foreclosed or ended (Antelius, 2007).

Other narratives that look towards a better future include a redemption sequence. Such narratives include a focus on personal actions, responsibility, and autonomy. A redemptive sequence is an important consideration for narratives that demonstrate how bad circumstances can be turned to good (McAdams et al., 2001). Importantly, these stories are associated with emotionally negative beginnings changing to emotionally positive endings; they identify with action and create purpose and meaning (Dunlop, 2022). In a redemptive sequence, the teller of the story illustrates how the negative aspects of life following an event (e.g., illness diagnosis) can be transformed into a better life scene. A common narrative that follows the onset of illness is termed the didactic narrative. This plot is focused on the need to search for and understand treatments that can create hope. Other master plots that demonstrate a redemptive sequence and highlight the action initiated by the individual include the heroic narrative or overcoming the monster; both narratives demonstrate an orientation towards actions taken that demonstrate how challenges are overcome. Overcoming the monster is valuable because it provides the illustration of a journey regarding experience where positive change was accomplish. The value of this narrative is that it is complete and can demonstrate valuable characteristic of an individual and provides an illustration of accomplishment, victory, and success. Examples of a monster (or challenge) identified by people with chronic illness have included mental illness, isolation, or problems identified during experience of health care that need fixing (Alawafi et al., 2022). These examples illustrate an important element of a redemptive story, which is that such stories are associated with prosocial behaviour (Dunlop, 2022). These stories have been shown to be the most valued or preferred stories of healthcare students following training (Alawafi et al., 2023). Redemptive stories aid perseverance the commitment an individual makes towards facing difficult circumstances (McAdams & Guo, 2015). Accessing examples of these narrative master plots will provide illustrations of the individual's accomplishments and character, and this will provide a way to establish the ability of the person to realise success in their present circumstances.

Narratives that embrace the present and future

Master plots that embrace the future and accommodate or seek to use the loss experienced include a supernatural narrative or quest story (Soundy et al., 2013). There are some experiences, expressions, and stories that show a transformative sequence, where the event in the past transformed the individual and value or meaning could be made from the change, rather than good being turned to bad or bad being turned to good. The goal of this plot is to reframe what has happened and to use it so the experience can have value. The quest story is valued by healthcare professionals for being realistic, positive, and able to achieve acceptance (Soundy et al., 2010). It can be frequently expressed in chronic illness; for instance, one sub-type of the quest, a quest memoir, which illustrates an openness to challenge and acceptance of the illness and the future, is frequently told by people who have had a stroke (France et al., 2013). One participant from the study by France illustrated this narrative by stating, *"This thing has happened to me. . . . I just want to get on with my life and . . . I can't turn the clock back. I've got what I've got, go and deal with it and run my life accordingly"* (p. 1653). The forms of quest are important to acknowledge as well as include the quest manifesto and the quest mythology. The quest manifest focuses on the need for social reform or social insight because of the insight gained from having an illness. The quest auto mythology identifies a rebirth, a change of character, or self-reinvention. These narratives narrative appears to highlight the ability to access important factors, which positively influence hope including drawing on characteristic of the self and finding new ways to establish meaning.

Table 5.1 A summary of the master plots and expressions of illness and how time is viewed.

Narrative Master plot	Past	Present	Future
Narratives that highlight a negative future, a downfall or limited future including the sad, tragic, detached, or chaotic narratives	Loss identified	Acceptance or chronic sorrow	Future based on present circumstances, that is limited or worst case non-existent. May be de-energised because of the loss
Narratives that observe or review events that have occurred including the comic or detached narratives	Loss or challenge to be understood	Acknowledgement with an openness to reconsider	Understood but to be re-represented and may be used to provide relief
Narratives that focus on a better future including the restitution (redemptive sequence)	Complete restoration	No acceptance	To be restored from the past. May rely on external support or intervention (like medicine) to be achieved
Narratives that focus on a better future including the didactic, heroic, or overcoming the monster	Problem identified and acknowledged	Problem or difficulty identified to be overcome	Create a better future from the present by overcoming the past. Energised and action orientated with more perception of control compared to other types
Narratives that embrace the present and future including the supernatural, adventure, or quest (transformative sequence)	Problem embraced and past acknowledged	Embrace what has happened move forward	To embrace the future a transformative view is needed. For instance, what has happened can be used and has a purpose

Key points

- Understanding the different master plots will help healthcare professionals understand when and if the patient is already using strategies that can aid hope.
- Healthcare professionals appear to react differently to specific narratives; following training a lack of empathy can be associated with the chaos

narrative, whilst the restitution narrative can be considered unrealistic or not accepting what has happened. Such response can infer negative characteristics of the teller.

- Stories that are redemptive appear to be more acceptable and valued following healthcare training, this implies being able to gain a fuller understanding of the individuals' life, and pre-illness may be important, and establishing information that reveals their character and ability to deal with situations may aid empathy from healthcare professionals.
- Because empathy was provided for overcoming the monster narrative, being able to understand how individuals have previously overcome challenges could be a useful way to enable hope to be developed.

Conclusion

The expression of illness through master plots is important as it provides individuals with an opportunity to convey their experience. It may be that specific settings, illnesses, or cultures tell similar plots. Being able to listen to the plot and allow the expression is an important task for healthcare professionals.

6 Introducing the model of emotions, adaptation, and hope (MEAH)

Introduction

Past models of hope are complicated and introduce a lot of concepts; for instance, Hasse et al. (1992) identify a process model around hope, which identifies several antecedents, attributes, and outcomes. Each of these aspects has multiple considerations. In a similar way, Herth (1990) identifies that the model proposed by Dufault and Maartocchio (1985) is complex and lacked testing. Further to this, past models of hope do not include and capture other essential elements of psychological reactions. For instance, psychological reactions to illness are captured as individually experienced psychodynamic reactions and represented by specific terms like anxiety, depression, denial, and anger (Livneh, 2022). These reactions build on the understanding of psychological adaptation in terms of stage or phase models. Past stage or phase models highlight singular words to describe adaptation, and this could include words that highlight the importance of acceptance or non-acceptance (denial), as well as key emotions (anger and depression) and shock (Smedema et al., 2009). Such models touch on concepts related to hopelessness by identifying despair or depression. However, the past models of adaptation do not integrate hope as part of the expression of adaptation despite hope being represented within experiences of chronic illness (Soundy et al., 2013). More recent considerations and updates to such models by Livneh (2022) consider a framework. This framework recognises hope, and it separates hope as an antecedent to the reaction and represents it as part of a contextual status. Other models that focus on the expression of illness can also be complicated and hard to follow and apply pragmatically. For instance, research in motor neurone disease (Soundy & Condon, 2015) describes the importance of the impact of an event on the different levels of hope, which flows to both initial reactions related to the expression of hope and hope-enabling responses as well as initial responses which disable hope, which should be considered within the context of the factors which influence hope. This is very much linked to cycles which enable or disable hope, something that has also been observed in Parkinson's disease (Soundy et al., 2014a). The past models all

DOI: 10.4324/9781003466161-6

have a limited ability for practical application due to the complexity of terms. A more simplified expression of adaptation was identified when considering the psychological properties of narrative master plots, and this identified that master plots of chronic illness contain an element of adaptation in the present, hope (or hopelessness) for the future, and an expression of emotions (e.g., Soundy et al., 2013; Soundy et al., 2014d). For instance, the restitution narrative represents an inability to accept the situation (adaptation), whilst using the past as a position to get back to in the future as a firm hope (complete or concrete hope). The importance and value of combining hope and adaptation as a simple scale (and the MEAH model) were recognised within a review considering individuals with multiple sclerosis (Soundy et al., 2016a).

The MEAH was created to capture emotions, psychological adaptation, and hope within a total of five questions. The idea of this is that an assessment or conversation is made quickly but is attentive to central aspects of psychological adaptation. The first question asks an individual to name what they are finding most difficult or challenging at that moment in time. This is important because from coping literature around the role of temporality (Lazarus, 1966), it can be identified that naming a challenge requires a future orientation which can be linked to feelings of hope (Livneh, 2015). Identifying a primary challenge also provides an opportunity to reveal what may prevent hope or the ability to accessing meaningful activities or relationships. After the challenge is identified, four questions are used to rate the challenge in terms of hope, psychological adaptation, and emotions (see Table 6.1). This model can be represented by two outcome measures, including the Hope and Adaptation Scale (Soundy et al., 2016b) and the circumplex model of affect (Russell, 1980). Figure 6.1 provides a basic image of the map identified by the MEAH. The MEAH considers a named challenge against how the hope for change, the ability to accept, the energy to deal with the challenge, and the feelings towards it.

The heart of the model is identified by the first three questions from the hope and adaptation scale (Soundy et al., 2016b). This scale provides the first three questions of the MEAH and provides a simple way to assess how adaptation and hope are expressed in relationship to a named challenge. The idea for the assessment of emotions comes from the circumplex model of affect provides a way to identify emotions and usefully considers energy and feelings. The first question (Q1) of the MEAH considers what challenge a patient is currently facing. The current version of the form words this question as follows: "What is the one aspect of your life right now that you are finding most difficult or challenging to adapt to?" This is followed by four questions (Q2-Q5; see Table 6.1) that have a guided response scale each with three options representing responses which illustrate a high, middle, or low response. Each response is accompanied by an emoji that represents a happy face (high), neural face (middle), or unhappy face (low). This version was designed to enable an interaction, whereas earlier and other versions may be more suitable if used as a screening tool.

Table 6.1 The 4 key guided response scale questions (Q2-Q5) from the MEAH (adapted from Soundy et al., 2023).

AREA	*Question*	*Response Scale*		
		Extreme high or complete response	*Middle or average response*	*Extreme Low, no ability or response which shows rejection*
Q2:Hope	How hopeful are you right now you can change this?	Completely hopeful 😄	Accept it may not be possible to change 🙂	See no hope or ability to change 🙁
Q3:Acceptance	To what extent are you able to accept this difficulty currently?	Completely able to embrace 😄	Can acknowledge it 🙂	Not able to accept and reject it 🙁
Q4: Energy	How much energy do you have to deal with this currently?	Very high energy 😄	Average energy 🙂	No energy 🙁
Q5: Feelings	How do you feel about it ranging from positive/ pleasant to negative/ unpleasant?	Extremely pleasant and positive feelings 😄	Average or normal feelings towards it 🙂	Extremely unpleasant and negative feelings 🙁

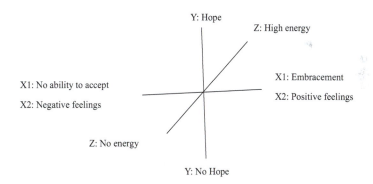

Figure 6.1 The idea of the MEAH as a map of psycho-emotional responses that help interpret a difficulty faced.

The first question of the MEAH tool is different from many other self-report outcome measures as it considers hope relative to a named difficulty, task, or challenge. This means the questions that follow provide a psychological response to a name difficulty, and if the scale is used more than once, it will consider each response as relative, and if used as a screening tool, it will be able to establish change with regard to that difficulty. Further to this, the identification of the challenge will provide an indication of what needs to be overcome and if the named difficulty could be a cause of suffering.

The final four questions provide capture a psycho-emotional response, which allows adaptation, hope, energy, and feelings to be mapped (see Figure 6.1, as an example of the map). This is important as hope, like different emotions are considered concepts which may be unpredictable and constantly changing. The changes experienced by individuals could be related to individuals, their context, time, or being part of groups (Pinto et al., 2023). Further consideration of hope and acceptance, as well as emotions, is needed to gain a greater understanding of the importance of these concepts. This detail is provided below.

Axis 1: hope and acceptance

Within the MEAH, both hope and acceptance are represented by two spectrums of responses. The ends of the spectrums and the middle of the spectrums are clearly identifiable and considered below for the terms, evidence, and information that helps identify the significance of the terms used within each spectrum.

The X1 axis of the MEAH: acceptance and the response to the present circumstance

The first spectrum considers how the individuals express adaptation to their present circumstances (see Figure 6.2). This can range from a complete embracement towards an inability to accept (also termed illness denial). The middle of the spectrum is identified as acknowledgement. Acknowledgement is an important stage of psychological adaptation because it represents the first indication that an individual has cognitively reconciled the condition, its permanence, and the future implications (Semdema et al., 2009). Acknowledgement provides recognition of the situation or some level of objectivity towards identifying how one is feeling, thinking, or behaving. This demonstrates a recognition that the challenges exist in the present circumstances, but an individual has not resigned themselves to a particular outcome (Soundy et al., 2016a).

Acceptance represents a stage towards embracement of the situation. Acceptance has been defined as "*a present-oriented activity requiring energy and characterized by receptivity toward and satisfaction with someone or something, including past circumstance, present situations, others and, ultimately, the* self" (Hasse et al., 1992, p. 144). It has long been considered an important part of psychological adaptation (Taylor, 1983). For instance, it is recognised that acceptance facilitates personal growth, a sense of self-worth, freedom, and some degree of self-transcendence (Hasse et al., 1992). It has also been identified at the point at which the chronic illness becomes part of

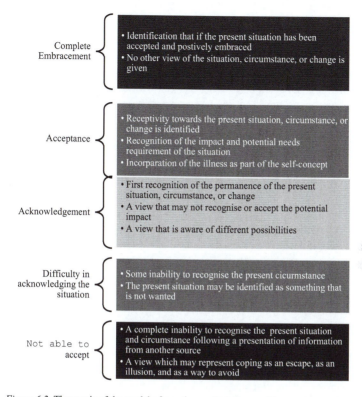

Figure 6.2 The x axis of the model of emotions, adaptation, and hope.

the individual's self-concept (Wright, 1983) and associated with the ability to pursue meaningful activities for people with chronic pain (McCracken et al., 2004).

In contrast, at the other end of the spectrum, denial has been identified as an individual having difficulty accepting, the nature, existence, or degree of impact of a condition or illness and should be understood in this context rather than identifying an individual as "in denial" (Kortte & Wegener, 2004; Rabinowitz & Peirson, 2006). To classify that illness denial is occurring, it is suggested that the patient needs to have received an adequate appraisal of the medical or diagnostic situation and details of its management with opportunity to clarify this and discuss it (Patiero et al., 2023).

Denial *post-illness* onset can have a psychologically protective function and can be seen as a reappraisal or recognition of reality to reduce realities associated with stress that are not wanted. Patiero et al. (2023) identify that post-illness denial can serve an adaptive function providing individual with time to process and dilute information that is distressing. It is also considered more beneficial following diagnosis or at the onset of disease and when used for shorter periods of time (Livneh, 2012). Protection against turmoil and stress can serve to aid adaptation to the situation at hand initially (Kortte & Wegener, 2004). It has been regarded as part of emotion focused coping the role of which is to help regulate emotional distress (Lazarus & Folkman, 1984), and it has been associated with a lower level of anxiety in certain illness populations and can be considered successful in managing stress (Livneh, 2012). However, the outcomes of denial, whether pre-illness or over a longer term, are problematic (Kortte & Wegener, 2004). For instance, denial may mean that emotional expressions are unresolved (De Ridder et al., 2008). Finally, different forms of denial have been identified within the coping literature like escape, avoidance, or wishful thinking. These types of denial have been associated with increased anxiety (Livneh, 2012).

The Y-axis of the MEAH: hope and the ability to look forward

Soundy et al. (2013, 2014, 2016) focus on the expression of hope within a spectrum (see Figure 6.3). The spectrum of hope represents an expression of hope existing from no hope to certain hope. The spectrum has significant points that need further consideration. The top part of the spectrum of hope may be broken down further into two important distinct views of hope. The first view is hope as an anticipation of event or outcome or the second as a want or desire for an outcome (Wiles et al., 2008). The first definition (hope as anticipation) may be distinguished as leading to a more certain outcome, perhaps with greater grounds for expecting the event or outcome (Stephenson, 1991). Emotions may link with this as more positive high or low-energy emotions (such as excitement or relief, respectively). It is important to note that what is hoped for is probable and that there is a desire around it (Smith, 2008); both (being probable and having desire) are subject to changing in intensity and time. Hope can exist without expectation although it cannot exist without desire (Stempsey, 2015). The second view of hope is as a desire; this seems to link more to feeling a sense of what is probable or an expectation beyond visible facts (Menninger, 1959), Put in another way having a greater chance than zero of achieving a goal (Stotland, 1969). To understand this further, an example of musculoskeletal trauma can be considered. A man with a simple fracture may anticipate that it gets better, whereas with more complex trauma, whilst anticipation may be there, events like multiple surgeries and having to wait to see the outcome of surgery make hope seem likely, but not anticipated. Another example could be following a stroke, where the outcome of mobility may be unknown; this in turn illustrates a more difficult and challenging situation to navigate. In the case of not knowing an outcome, healthcare professionals and patients may draw back on the

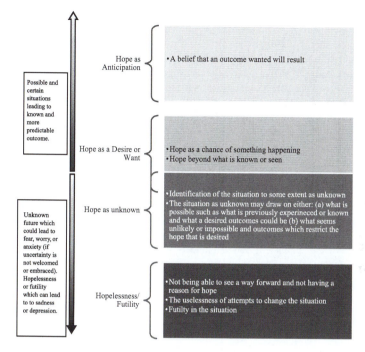

Figure 6.3 The y-axis of the model of emotions, adaptation, and hope.

idea of what is realistic, known or previously experienced, or use examples of what happened to others.

Within the middle of the spectrum and in situations where the certainty of an outcome is not known, hope can be identified by considering what is possible. Soundy et al. (2013) state that hope in possibility can represent a point where an individual has been able to reconcile their present circumstances with what the future may be. This suggests an openness to change and an acceptance of the unknown and generates access to hope as a desire. In chronic illness, where hope in possibility relates to the ability to change a situation or circumstance, it is very easy to be aware that, as much as change may be possible, it may also be impossible. Lazarus (1999) links hope in possibility with a certain known anxiety; as such, we need to be aware of the emotions that connect with hope, especially when what is hoped for is unknown.

Within the middle of the spectrum, but below possibility, is where uncertainty sits. Uncertainty is closely linked to possibility. The central aspects of uncertainty include the inability to assign a definite value to objects and events or not being able to accurately predict outcomes (Mishel, 1988). Uncertainty is identified as a major barrier to future-related conversations, especially in end-of-life care (Momen et al., 2012). As such, an individual can consider many different outcomes or diverse evaluations or conclusions. Uncertainty and unknown situations are likely to occur before what is possible is identified and therefore is an important factor that influences psychological adaptation. Uncertainty can be experienced where either a desired repsonse or an undesired reponse to an event can be expressed (Mishel, 1990).

Where circumstances illustrate an outcome to be less likely or impossible, unless that desire can be changed, adapted, or reframed, it is likely to lead to no hope or futility. The idea of hopelessness is identified by Lynch (1965) as containing three central aspects: first is a lack of feeling or value in attempting change, second there is a sense of things feeling too-much, and finally there is an identification that what is hoped for is impossible. Given this definition, it is easy to see how this construct is heavily emotive and allows little distance to objectively consider the situation. Hopelessness is directly related to experience and change and knowledge, but it is also related to how uncertain the future appears (Soundy et al., 2013). It has been described in coping literature as representing the direct opposite of being able to cope because all responses an individual gives will lead to a negative result (Ursin & Eriksen, 2003).

Axis 2 emotions: energy and feelings

Emotions have been defined as *"neural circuits (that are at least partially dedicated), response systems and a feeling state/process that motivates and organises cognition and action"* (Izard, 2010, p. 367). Emotions include psychological states and are central to psychological models of the human mind (Gross & Barrett, 2011). Emotions have been identified as a state which is represented by a feeling (i.e., a sensation with a valence) and a motivation (i.e., an action tendency) that drives behaviour (Finan et al., 2011). Emotions are reflected in physiological arousal, behavioural expression, and subjective experiences; they prepare an organism to act or response to the environmental demands (Leverson, 1994). Simpson (2004) identifies that hope fits best within a theoretical framework that recognises the multi-dimension features of emotions. Emotions are considered important because they reveal the individual's response to situations and events, which are often outside their own control, are connected to relationship with others, and can reveal our beliefs and judgements. The acknowledgement and processing of emotions are generally identified as valuable for psychological adjustment, whilst the uncontrolled expression of emotions can be maladaptive (de Ridder et al., 2008; Gratz & Roemer, 2004). Emotions can be important to understand the context of pain and suffering. For instance, negative emotions may be amplified during pain catastrophising; however, positive emotions appear to buffer individual reactivity to pain (Sturgeon & Zautra, 2013). Further to this, people with higher levels of hope identify higher intensities of positive emotions more frequently, as well as less intense and fewer negative emotions (Synder et al., 1991).

When individuals are hopeful, they are more positive. Positive emotions have also been associated with a greater ability to problem solve and identify meaningful goals (Ciarrochi et al., 2015). Intervention studies have identified that postive emotional expressions are assoicated with improved psycholgoical and physical adjustment and improved disease activity (de Ridder et al., 2008).

The measurement of emotions has a long history of consideration, beyond the scope of this book. Within the MEAH, emotions are captured using the circumplex model of affect (Russell, 1980). See Figure 6.3 via the x-z axis. This is important because this model of affect can identify a range of emotions but also links to specific types of emotional coping (the identification of how people regulate emotions under stress). Positive emotional coping is associated with low arousal or energy and high valence of positive feelings, and negative emotional coping is linked to high-energy states with negative valence or negative feelings about what is happening (Stanislawski, 2019). The ability to recognise emotions is important for people with chronic illness. For instance, individuals with chronic illness can be less effective at managing emotional regulation that this can predict the inability to access meaningful relationships and negative impact quality of life (Cooper et al., 2014). Further to this, the inability to identify and articulate emotions is associated with greater distress for people with chronic illness (Schmidt & Andrykowski, 2004).

When we consider suffering, one way to gain a deep understanding of specific emotions is to use scales, which can identify different individual responses. The circumplex model of affect is ideal for identifying specific emotions (Russell, 1980; Soundy et al., 2016a). This is important because specific emotions can have consequences for individuals (Leverson, 1994). For instance, anger has been associated with increased cardiovascular symptoms in individuals following observations of the emotions during a 20-year longitudinal cohort study (Leverson & Gottman, 1983). Emotional turmoil or ambivalence can accompany traumatic events. For instance, processing of events for the first time can be accompanied by mourning, depression, shock, or anger (Smedema et al., 2009). Emotions are created as the change is interpreted, hope and fear can present at the same time, and hopes could be engulfed by negative emotions and worries. Worries could be of not living, of future complications (Leite et al., 2021). Hope and fear are interconnected, and addressing fears is important for healthcare professionals (Parker-Oliver, 2002). Fear can often be associated with loss of independence and autonomy caused by a chronic illness (Pinto et al., 2023). In a similar way, hope and negative emotions like sadness are also interconnected. For instance, negative affect has been associated with decreasing hope, but increasing hope decreases negative affect (Ciarrochi et al., 2015).

One critical question within the MEAH tool is the assessment of energy. Energy is acknowledged as an essential component of psychosocial adaptation to chronic illness, trauma, and disability (Livneh, 2022) and is particularly important to understand. For instance, boredom and a perception of fatigue can act together to prevent engaging behaviours and divert or redirect behaviour to other activities (Inzlicht et al., 2018). Individuals need to have the energy to accept and self-transcend circumstances, which are attributes closely associated with hope (Hasse et al., 1992). The experience of fatigue, in turn, can mean there is limited energy that can be used for hope (Herth, 1990). Mental fatigue has been identified as tiredness and exhaustion, an aversion to continue with activities, and a decreased level of commitment to the task being performed (Boksem & Tops, 2008). Mental fatigue is associated with changes in behaviour, mood, and the ability to process information (Desmond & Handcock, 2001), and it significantly and negatively affects planning, adaptation, and attention in a negative way (Boksem & Tops, 2008).

Fatigue and a lack of energy can be linked to a disease and physical pain, but fatigue should also be considered in terms of mental tiredness. For instance, extreme tiredness is associated with the experience of rheumatic disease and pain, but also mental tiredness results from not understanding it fully (Sällfors et al., 2002). Another consideration is that uncertainty produces high arousal (Ursin & Eriksen, 2004), and uncertainty is especially important to understand and is interlinked with hope. The circumplex model can be understood as being arranged into six clusters of responses (Carroll et al., 1999), where the each axis (x2 axis and z axis) are arranged into positive reactions (high energy, e.g., excited/thrilled; medium energy, e.g., happy/pleased; or low energy, e.g., calm/peaceful) and negative reactions (high energy, e.g., tense/distressed; medium energy, e.g., unhappy/displeased; or low energy, e.g., lethargic/depressed). Further different emotions can be identified by combing the different emotions, which are identified by a linear combination of the two axis (Posner et al., 2005). It is beyond the scope of this work to consider a more detailed critique of this model as presented in the literature. However, it is clear it has pragmatic value for understanding and distinguishing emotions in a brief way for a targeted challenge as required by the MEAH.

Interaction between concepts

There is a clear interaction between the concepts and axis of hope, acceptance, and emotions (energy and feelings). Research has associated acceptance (x1 axis) to other concepts. For instance, the first stage or recognition of present circumstance (acknowledgement) is regarded as an essential stimulus for hope when an individual is suffering (Miller, 2007). The value of acceptance has been further considered. For instance, acceptance is identified as providing a resolution to fear associated with an unwanted experience (Hasse et al., 1992). Acceptance also allows a release of engery once required for resistance against that which was not wanted and once achieved it enhances the individual's ability to be receptive to situations about oneself or others, it enables an individual to feel satisfied, it has a focus on the present circumstances and enables self-acceptance. Acceptance requires further consideration in its association with hope. For instance, accepting what is happening does not mean giving up and does not mean that the individual must change their view of hope, so in having hope, there is also a non-acceptance, which is not a revolt or denial (Marcel, 1951). This non-acceptance can be considered as agency to move forward or a way to transcend the circumstances (Barnard, 1995). However, the balance in hope may be regarded as the need to both accept limitations when looking forward but to want to defy limitations to allow the creation of possibility. Something Barnard (1995) refers to as the paradox of hope. The complexity of the association between the hope spectrum and acceptance axis is complicated further when denial is considered. For instance, denial has a negative association to optimism in people with multiple sclerosis (Livneh, 2009). Other research has identified what could be considered common-sense responses around hope. For instance, the perceived expectancy within hope can be directly related to an emotional response. For instance, Ursin and Eriksen (2004) identified that if an outcome that is not wanted is perceived as (a) highly likely, this can lead to high arousal and fear; (b) unknown, this can lead to high arousal but anxiety; or (c) unlikely, this can lead to low arousal and feelings of safety. Further understanding of this interaction is important. One way to do this is by using common story plots (Soundy et al., 2014d), and each plot appears to combine the hope and acceptance axis differently. It may ultimately be easier to work with and understand stories from a pragmatic perspective, and storytelling research appears to have positive psycho-emotional benefits (Bryne & Soundy, 2020).

In addition to these interactions, it is important to acknowledge that a challenge experienced by an individual will be influenced by other factors identified in Chapters 3 and 4, including psychological, social, and environmental (Soundy et al., 2014c). Each of these factors may explain the ability to be hopeful and find meaning as an individual looks forward. Once meaningful goals can be identified, and suffering understood and an adequate distance gained from events which cause suffering, it is more possible and probable that an individual can access a motivated state needed for particularised hope to be achieved. That is, the ability to gain access to particularised hopes cannot be taken for granted and require support. The next chapter considers how understanding the factors which influence hope can be integrated into a conversation as an extended version of the tool.

Key points

- The MEAH captures a response to challenge that identifies psychological (adaptation and hope) and emotional map of that response.
- The importance of capturing a range of emotions and hope is important because of how quickly both can change and how they can respond to an experience of being heard.

- Being able to investigate energy is important to understand how physical and mental fatigue may impact the individual and their response to a challenge that is faced.
- Establishing emotions is important because of the ability to change. However, repeated and prolonged consideration and focus on negative emotions or rumination on them may be less valuable (de Ridder et al., 2008).

Conclusion

Understanding that the challenges people face can be expressed via different components of psychological adaptation is important and being able to name these components including hope, adaptation, feelings, and energy provides a way to map a response. The hope and adaptation scale may be particularly important in being able to successfully support hope.

7 Introducing the application and findings of the MEAH within clinical practice

Introduction

The past chapter has identified a tool that considers brief questions to assess a primary challenge faced by patients (Soundy et al., 2016a, 2016b). The advantage of the tool is that it provides a broad assessment of psychological adaptation, hope, and emotions. Concepts which are linked together and can be understood to represent how able an individual is to look forward, to embrace what has happened in the present and how they feel about the challenge and how much energy they must access. The tool can be used in three ways: as a screening tool, as a brief tool that enables a hope entered conversation, or as an extended version allowing for a greater consideration of the key factors that influence hope. There have been two principal applications of the MEAH within clinical training and practice. This has included (a) as a scale and short therapeutic encounter and (b) as an extended therapeutic interaction towards developing goals.

As a scale and short encounter

The first use of the MEAH tool was as a scale and supportive interaction. The first application of the tool was during the COVID-19 lockdown to support physiotherapy students (Soundy et al., 2021a). This demonstrated the responsiveness of the scale to being able to talk about a difficulty and rate it. The work highlighted the value of using a scale in an online environment. Results identified positive changes in hope, acceptance, energy, and feelings following a short 10-minute interaction. The work highlighted the value of a meaningful interaction that focused on a named difficulty and subsequent questions. The idea of this work supported the need to understand and identify a named difficulty. The focus on difficulty and being able to consider it in relationship to hope, adaptation, energy, and feelings helped individuals to positively change how they considered and felt about the difficulty. This work highlighted how quickly hope and emotions can change and respond to being listened to and paved a way for further development of the MEAH tool. Following this training, healthcare professionals and students were taught to use the tool. An experimental study

DOI: 10.4324/9781003466161-7

(Soundy et al., 2021b) initially compared the benefits of brief training for students. A single training session of either the MEAH brief tool or motivational interviewing training was provided to randomly assigned physiotherapy students. Positive results were identified for both groups, including increases in self-efficacy (confidence) and communication. The MEAH training, however, appeared to help students perceive that they would be able to manage distressing communication more effectively compared to the motivational interviewing group. This provided the opportunity to further develop the training and enhance it with the use of simulated practice (Soundy et al., 2024). This study considered a stroke scenario and reported significant learning points for training: Students identified that before the simulated practice, there was a belief among students that applying the MEAH was straightforward. However, following the interaction, challenges were identified by students. One need was identified as a need to have a deeper understanding of background of the psychological and emotional components of the MEAH. All students valued the brief training and simulated practice. The practical nature of the simulated experience was identified as having value because it provided a safe space for developing the interaction. Simulated practice was identified as being valuable before placements or near them for the best application of practice. The practical experience provided the students with experience on how to overcome difficulties during conversations. Differences between the online application of the MEAH and the in-person application of the MEAH were identified. The in-person interaction was identified as more challenging by students; one main reason for this appeared to be the non-verbal communication that required additional attention. Following the development of the training and simulated practice, the MEAH was developed for a research placement for students. Students were required to test the tool and develop a research paper around their experiences of applying the tool for people with stroke. Submissions from students from the placement identified that the MEAH provided a deeper understanding of the experiences of people with stroke compared to normal clinical questions and encounters. It allowed students to identify a primary difficulty (e.g., the most frequently identified challenges included an inability to walk or difficulty with walking, body weakness, or speech problems); it allowed people with stroke to talk to students about their needs and help students develop empathy during the interaction.

As an extended encounter

The most recent placement of the MEAH (Soundy et al., 2023) tested an extended version that incorporates other elements of hope identified within this book. The extended version of the tool looks to consider three further areas after the initial questions. This includes: (a) exploring the difficulty further by considering how it has changed across time, its impact on roles, social identities, activity participation, and functioning; (b) how the difficulty can be helped by considering factors that aid hope with questions around activities, cognitive strategies, and support or inspiration from peers; and (c) the identification of goals based on what the patient believes could help with the difficulty, as well as identifying pathways that would help achieve the goals. During the application of the extended version trained physiotherapy students (Soundy et al., 2023) delivered the intervention and identified that 11 people could identify a goal and 6 did not. Most people with stroke (n = 5/6) of those who didn't have a goal identified a low level of hope, whilst most often in the goal group a high level of hope was identified (n = 5/11). It was identified that some people with stroke in the goal group experienced deterioration over time (n = 3/11) and over half (n = 6/11) identified the need to focus on managing their difficulty. Whereas half (n = 3/5) of the people with stroke in the no goal group identified no perceived change over time.

It is important to note that the value of the interaction doesn't hinge on identifying a goal, as in this recent work several people with stroke didn't identify a goal but still reported benefits of the interaction and being heard. For those who did identify a goal, it is possible that specific goal frameworks (Scobbie et al., 2020) or aspects of hope therapy (Cheavens & Guter, 2018) interactions could provide a way to move the interaction forward. For instance, this could include strategies that enhance energy (like physical activity, diet, and sleep). The extended conversations were identified as beneficial because the conversations identified some aspects of their life they had not talked about for a while and considered feelings and expression of their own view. The questions and ability to listen to the answers from people with stroke were valued, notably the lack of interruptions to answers given. The no-goal group valued talking about challenges even though no goal was identified. Goal-directed behaviour may result from two forms of motivation: the need to avoid harm/punishment or further suffering or the motivation for the need to achieve rewards. Both are associated with a cost to an individual's energy, people are more likely to expend energy when the expenditure is perceived as low against a reward which is considered high (Boksem & Tops, 2008). Understanding rewards and costs of behaviour is fundamental to all goals identified (Miller, 2000), and being able to identify attainable goals can promote positive emotions (Helegson & Zajdel, 2017); the above reasons may help explain why those with a poorer prognosis in this study identified goals more frequently. In other words, the use and value of hope are needed more when greater challenges are perceived.

Some individuals with stroke, when considering the extended version of the MEAH tool (Soundy et al., 2023), identified the value of the work in hospital or at discharge, and two individuals cautioned about using it straight after a stroke and identified that some time was needed to be able to correctly respond. Further work needs to consider how and when to consider using the extended tool. The students who were trained to deliver the MEAH most often identified the benefit and importance of talking to others in a specific and structured way. The extended tool provided time to consider the experiences and feelings of people with stroke. This was identified as important and contrasted against a typical clinical placement experience.

The application of the tool in practice has used varied approaches, including following questions exactly to understanding principles and asking questions that are related to the concepts identified by the MEAH. Further to the above, ideas from the work can be taken forward. For example, it may be that, following reading this book, additional questions that consider key or critical emotions that have affected individuals across time or most consistently or factors which may be most influential on energy are considered within clinical practice. Healthcare professionals may also benefit from considering how individuals can look forward. This may include questions around how patients consider rehabilitation is going and being experienced, what is expected as they look forward, or understanding how they perceive themselves as learning new functioning and viewing experiences in different ways. Further, as rehabilitation progresses, considering how the application of the MEAH is in different environments and settings would be useful.

Key points

- Simulated practice is important for understanding how to apply the tool, and practical experience is essential to develop conversations using the MEAH.
- The online application of the MEAH was experienced in a more straight-forward way with less difficulties compared to an in-person interaction in a simulated scenario.
- The tool is identified as valuable for a meaningful interaction that can identify a patient's situation and challenges, feelings and emotions which in turn helps develop empathy.
- Therapists should consider the ability to express how someone is feeling as a good outcome regardless of the ability to identify a goal, as this is important to positive and hopeful interactions.
- The MEAH tool may be particularly important at points of change like discharge, where change will be experienced to understand the impact of that change.
- The responses to the MEAH may provide a precursor to more serious clinical mood disorders.
- For individuals who identify a goal following an extended interaction with the MEAH, there may be value in supplementing this with a framework related to goal setting.

Conclusion

The development of the MEAH tool has been identified as having value for healthcare professionals and students who have been trained as well as patients who receive the tool. The extended version uses more questions that consider factors that influence hope as identified in earlier chapters. One central need that was expressed as part of the training was that of practice in a simulated environment to understand the application of the tool and to receive feedback and reflect on how the tool is used. Further research is needed into the application of the tool to broader groups.

8 Conclusions

Conclusions

This book provides a focus on the importance and role of hope for people with chronic illness and identifies how hope can be harnessed. Whilst writing this book, three specific points stood out that are worthy of being mentioned again here. First, uncertainty, although often considered in a negative light has instances when it can be experienced differently and some people with chronic illness can seek it out and see it as part of an adventure. Second, false hope as perceived by a patient, parent, or spouse may have a psychologically protective role. It may be expressed initially, following an event trauma or challenge, or following change. Healthcare professionals and others who look to "correct" false hope should only do so when other hopes have been established. Remembering that false hope is better than no hope, and there are times when a non-acceptance of a situation has value, for instance because it is associated with greater agency. A danger for healthcare professionals is that they introduce false despair by denying a patients hope, and this should be avoided.

The work addressed the challenges faced by healthcare professionals by considering how conversations about the future can be undertaken. Several specific points from this book are worth of mention within this chapter. First, the MEAH as well as the extended version of the MEAH provides a useful brief interaction tool for healthcare professionals. It is critical that healthcare professionals are made aware of the key components of the MEAH, most importantly hope, adaptation, and energy, and understand that exploring each of these aspects around a challenge will provide insight to the well-being of the patient and allow for a meaningful interaction to occur. Second, it is also important that healthcare professionals are aware of the levels of hope. This includes the expression of suffering, the meaning found in relationships and activities, and social roles patients have. Time will not be wasted by exploring these aspects during an interaction. Third, it is important that healthcare professionals consider how time is used and if and how patients can look forward. Where and if the future does not seem possible, healthcare professionals may

DOI: 10.4324/9781003466161-8

benefit from being able to explore and find different possibilities that exist and can be found within the different levels of hope expressed by a patient. Finally, illness narrative master plots may represent an easy way to capture a psychological response as well as a view and focus on time from a patient. Being aware of master plots within specific cultural setting and being able to offer other stories provide one useful way of supporting patients through interaction in a non-directive way.

Healthcare professionals will benefit from the development of brief and effective psychological tools that are easy to remember and apply in clinical practice. The value of the MEAH is that it can be learnt quickly and be provided during brief interactions over a single session. The initial results from training and applying the MEAH in clinical practice demonstrate the efficacy of the approach and the importance of understanding the primary challenges people face and being able to explore this is valuable. The verbalisation of such challenges provides useful ground to establish therapeutic relationships and explore how the identified challenge can be overcome and the individual supported in the most appropriate way. People often expressed difficulties and psychological well-being through stories, being able to use and work with stories in clinical practice is highly valuable. The MEAH is also able to help healthcare professionals identify how the future is viewed using stories and consider how stories may be a device that can be used to support patients further.

References

Alawafi R, Rosewilliam S, Soundy A. (2022). A qualitative study of illness narratives: 'Overcoming the monster' master plot for patients with stroke. International Journal of Therapy and Rehabilitation, 29; 1–12.

Alawafi R, Rosewilliam S, Soundy A. (2023). Overcoming the monster! Perceptions of physiotherapy students regarding the use of stroke master plots for building therapeutic relationships; A vignette study. BMC Medical Education, 23; 311.

Anderson EC, Carleton RN, Diefenbach M, Han PKJ. (2019). The relationship between uncertainty and affect. Frontiers in Psychology, 10; 2504.

Antelius E. (2007). The meaning of the present: Hope and foreclosure in narrations about people with severe brain damage. Medical Anthropology Quarterly, 21; 324–342.

Apóstolo JL, Viveiros CS, Nunes HI, Domingues HR. (2007). Illness uncertainty and treatment motivation in type 2 diabetes patients. Revista latino-americana de enfermagem, 15; 575–582.

Barnard D. (1995). Chronic illness and the dynamics of hoping. In S.K. Toombs, D. Barnard, & R.A. Carson (Eds.), Chronic illness from experience to policy (pp. 38–57). Indiana University Press.

Block RA. (1990). Introduction. In RA Block (Ed.), Cognitive models of psychological time (pp. xiii–xix). Hillsdale, NJ: Lawrence Erlbaum Associates.

Boksem MAS, Tops M. (2008). Mental fatigue: Cost and benefits. Brain Research Reviews, 59; 125–139.

Boniwell I, Zimbardo PG. (2004). Balancing time perspective in pursuit of optimal functioning. In PA Linley & S Joseph (Eds.), Positive psychology in practice (pp. 165–178). John Wiley & Sons, Inc.

Bright FAS, Kayes NM, McCann CM, & McPherson KM. (2011). Understanding hope after stroke: A systematic review of the literature using concept analysis. *Topics in Stroke Rehabilitation*, 18(5); 490–508. https://doi.org/10.1310/tsr1805–490

Bright FAS, McCann CM, Kayes NM. (2019). Recalibrating hope: A longitudinal study of the experiences of people with aphasia after stroke. Scandinavian Journal of Caring Sciences, 34; 428–435.

Bright FAS, Soundy A, Madyak J, Kayes N. (2024). Limited conversations about constrained futures: Exploring clinicians' conversations about life after stroke in inpatient settings. Brain Impairment, 25; IB23067.

Brown P, de Graaf S. (2013). 'Considering a future which may not exist: The construction of time and expectations amidst advanced-stage cancer. Health, Risk & Society, 15; 543–560.

Brown P. (2011). The dark side of hope and trust: Constructed expectations and the value-for-money regulation of new medicines. Health Sociology Review, 20(4); 410–422.

Bryne C, Soundy A. (2020). The use of storytelling intervention for the promotion of physical activity in chronically ill patients: An integrative review. Physiotherapy, 27; 1–13.

Bueno-Gómez N. (2017). Conceptualising suffering and pain. Philosophy, Ethics and Humanities in Medicine, 12; 17. https://doi.org/10.1186/s13010-017-0049-5

Carleton RN. (2016). Into the unknown: A review and synthesis of contemporary models involving uncertainty. Journal of Anxiety Disorder, 39; 30–43.

Carroll JM, Yik MS, Russell JA, Feldman Barrett K. (1999). On the psychometric principles of affect. Review of General Psychology, 3; 14–22.

Cassel EJ. (2004). The nature of suffering and the goals of medicine. Oxford: Oxford University Press.

Charmaz K. (1983). Loss of self: A fundamental form of suffering in the chronically ill. Sociology of Health and Illness, 5; 169–195.

Cheavens JS, Whitted WM. (2023). Hope therapy. Current Opinion in Psychology, 49; 101509. doi: 10.1016/j.copsyc.2022.101509. Epub 2022 Nov 3. PMID: 36495712.

Cheavens, J. S., & Guter, M. M. (2018). Hope therapy. In M. W. Gallagher & S. J. Lopez (Eds.), The Oxford handbook of hope (pp. 133–142). Oxford University Press.

Ciarrochi J, Parker P, Kashdan TB, Heaven PCL, Barkus K. (2015). Hope and emotional well-being: A six-year study to distinguish antecedents, correlates and consequences. The Journal of Positive Psychology, 10; 520–532.

Colla R, Williams P, Oades LG, Camacho-Morles J. (2022). "A new hope" for positive psychology: A dynamics systems reconceptualization of hope theory. Frontiers in Psychology, 13; 1–15.

Conway MF, Pantaleao A, Popp JM. (2017). Parents' experience of hope when their child has cancer: Perceived meaning and the influence of health care professionals. Journal of Oncology Nursing, 34; 427–434.

Cooper CL, Phillips LH, Johnston M, Whyte M, MacLeod MJ. (2014). The role of emotion regulation on social participation following stroke. *British Journal of Clinical Psychology*, 54; 181–199. https://doi.org/10.1111/bjc.12068

Cross A, Schneider M. (2010). A preliminary qualitative analysis of the impact of hope on stroke recovery in women. Topics in Stroke Rehabilitation, 17; 484–495.

Cutliffe JR, Herth K. (2002). The concept of hope in nursing 1: Its origins, background and nature. British Journal of Nursing, 11; 832–840.

David D, Montgomery GH, Stan R, Dilorenzo T, Erblich J. (2004). Discrimination between hopes and expectancies for nonvolitional outcomes: Psychological phenomenon or artifact? Personality and Individual Differences, 36; 1945–1952.

De Graaf S. (2016). The construction and use of hope within health-settings: Recent developments in qualitative research and ethnographic studies. Sociology Compass, 10/7; 603–612. https://doi.org/10.1111/soc4.12380

De Ridder D, Geenen R, Kuijer R, van Middendorp H. (2008). Psychological adjustment to chronic disease. Lancet, 372; 246–255.

Declercq D, Kafle E, Peters J, Raby S, Chawner D, Blease J, Foye U. (2024). "Finding light in the darkness": Exploring comedy as an intervention for eating disorder recovery. Mental Health Review Journal, 29; 110–126.

Desmond PA, Hancock PA. (2001). Active and passive fatigue states. In PA Desmond & PA Hancock (Eds.), Stress, workload and fatigue (pp. 455–465). Mahwah, NJ: Lawrence Erlbaum Associates.

Dosedlová J, Jelínek M, Klimusová H, Burešová I. (2016). Positive expectations – optimism and hope in models. The European Proceedings of Social and Behavioural Sciences. Published from the ICEEPSY 2016: 7th International Conference on Education and Educational Psychology, 436–447.

Dufault KJ, Martocchio B. (1985). Hope: Its spheres and dimensions. The Nursing Clinics of North America, 20; 379–391.

Dunlop WL. (2022). The cycle of life and story: Redemptive autobiographical narratives and prosocial behaviours. Current Opinion in Psychology, 43; 213–218.

Ebright PR, Lyon B. (2002). Understanding hope and factors that enhance hope in women with breast cancer. Oncology Nursing Forum, 29(3):561–8. doi: 10.1188/02.ONF.561–568.

Elliott J. (Ed.). (2005). Using narrative in social research – Qualitative and quantitative approaches. Thousand Oaks, CA: SAGE.

Ersek M. (1992). The process of maintaining hope in adults undergoing bone marrow transplantation for Leukaemia. Oncology Nursing Forum, 19; 883–889.

Farran, C. J., Herth, K. A., & Popovich, J. M. (1995). Hope and hopelessness: Critical clinical constructs. Sage Publications, Inc.

Farran CJ, McCann J. (1989) Longitudinal analysis of hope in community-based older adults. *Archieves of Pscyhiatric nursing*, 3; 272–276.

Farran CJ, Herth K, Popovich J. (1995). Hope and hopelessness: Critical clinical constructs. Thousand Oaks, CA: SAGE.

Farran CJ, Popovich J. (1990). Hope: A relevant concept for geriatric psychiatry. Archives of Psychiatric Nursing, 4; 124–130.

Finan PH, Zautra AJ, Wershba R. (2011). Chapter 16. The dynamics of emotion in adaptation to stress. In R Contrada & A Baum (Eds.), The handbook of stress science: Biology, psychology and health. New York: Springer Nature.

Fong TCT, Lo TLT, Ho RTH. (2022). Indirect effects of social support and hope on quality of life via emotional distress among stroke survivors: A three-wave structural equation model. Frontiers in Psychiatry, 13; 919078.

France EF, Hunt K, Dow C, Wyke S. (2013). Do Men's and Women's Accounts of Surviving a Stroke Conform to Frank's Narrative Genres? Qualitative Health Research, 12; 1649–1659. Doi:10.1177/1049732313509895

French, T. M. (1952). The Integration of Behaviour. Chicago, IL: University of Chicago Press.

Frankl VE. (2004). Man's search for meaning. London: Penguin.

Gardenhire J, Mullet N, Fife S. (2019). Living with Parkinson's: The process of finding optimism. Qualitative Health Research, 29; 1781–1793.

Gergen KJ, Gergen MM. (1997). Narrative and the self as relationship. Advances in Experimental Social Psychology, 21; 17–56.

Gibson, J. (2017). A relational approach to suffering: A reappraisal of suffering in the helping relationship. Journal of Humanistic Psychology, 57(3), 281–300. https://doi.org/10.1177/0022167815613203

Goodman F, Disabato D, Kashdan T, Machell K. (2017). Personality strengths as resilience: A one-year multi-wave study. Journal of Personality, 85; 423–434.

Gorman BS, Wessman AE. (1977). Images, values and concepts of time in psychological research. In BS Gorman & AE Wessman (Eds.), The personal experience of time. New York: Plenum Press.

Gratz KL, Roemer L. (2004). Multidimensional assessment of emotion regulation and dysregulation: Development, factor structure and initial validation of the Difficulties in Emotion Regulation Scale. Journal of Psychopathology and Behavioural Assessment, 26; 41–54.

Gross JJ, Barrett LF. (2011). Emotion generation and emotion regulation: One or two depends on your point of view. Emotion Review, 3; 8–16.

Gum AM. (2017). Promoting hope in older adults. In MW Gallagher & SJ Lopez (Eds.), The Oxford handbook of hope (Vol. 1, pp. 143–155). Oxford: Oxford University Press.

Haahr A, Kirkevold M, Hall EOZ, Østergaard K. (2011). Living with advanced Parkinson's disease: A constant struggle with unpredictability. Journal of Advanced Nursing, 67; 408–417. https://doi.org/10.1111/j.1365-2648.2010.05459.x

Hammer K, Mogensen O, Hall EOC. (2009). The meaning of hope in nursing research: A meta-synthesis. Scandinavian Journal of Caring Sciences, 23; 549–557.

Hardcastle SJ, Hancox J, Hattar A, Maxwell-Smith C, Thøgersen-Ntoumani C, Hagger MS. (2015). Motivating the unmotivated: How can health behaviour be changed in those unwilling to change? Frontiers in Psychology, 6; 835.

Hasse J, Britt R, Coward D, Leidy N, Penn P. (1992). Simultaneous concept analysis of spiritual perspective, hope, acceptance and self-transcendence. Image: Journal of Nursing Scholarship, 24; 141–147.

Hayes L, Herrman H, Castle D, Harvey C. (2017). Hope, recovery and symptoms: The importance of hope for people living with severe mental illness. Australasian Psychiatry, 25; 583–587.

Haythornthwaite JA, Menefee LA, Heinberg LJ, Clark MR. (1998). Pain coping strategies predict perceived control over pain. Pain, 77; 33–39.

Helgeson VS, Zajdel M. (2017). Adjusting to chronic health conditions. The Annual Review of Psychology, 68; 545–571.

Herrestad H, Biong S, McCormack B, Borg M, Karlsson B. (2014). A pragmatist approach to the hope discourse in health care research. Nursing Philosophy, 15; 211–220.

Herth KA. (1992). Fostering hope in the terminally ill. Nursing Sciences Quarterly, 4; 177–184.

Herth KA. (1992). An abbreviated instrument to measure hope: Development and psychometric evaluation. Journal of Advanced Nursing, 17; 1251–1259.

Herth KA. (1993). Hope in the family caregiver of terminally ill people. Journal of Advanced Nursing, 18(4); 538–548.

Herth KA. (1995). Engendering hope in the chronically and terminally ill: Nursing interventions. American Journal of Hospice and Palliative Medicine, 12; 31–39.

Hill DL, Boyden JY, Feudtner C. (2023). Hope in the context of life-threatening illness and the end of life. Current Opinion in Psychology, 49; 101513.

Hinton D, Kirk S. (2017). Living with uncertainty and hope: A qualitative study exploring parents' experiences of living with childhood multiple sclerosis. Chronic Illness, 13; 88–99. doi: 10.1177/1742395316664959

Hockey GRJ. (2011). A motivational control theory of cognitive fatigue. In PL Ackerman (Ed.), Cognitive fatigue: Multidisciplinary perspectives on current research and future applications (pp. 167–188). Washington, DC: American Psychological Association.

Holdcraft C, Williamson C. (1991). Assessment of hope in psychiatric and chemically dependent patients. Applied Nursing Research, 4; 129–134.

Hume D. (1978). Treatise on human nature (2nd ed.). Edited by P Nidditch. Oxford: Oxford University Press.

Inzlicht M, Schmeichel BJ, Macrae CN. (2018). Why self-control seems (but may not be) limited. Trends in Cognitive Science, 18; 127–133.

Izard CE. (2010). The many meanings/aspects of emotion: Definitions, functions, activation and regulation. Emotion Review, 2; 363–370.

Javier-Aliaga DJ, Quispe G, Quineteros-Zuniga D, Adriano-Rengifo CE, White M. (2022). Hope and resilience related to fear of COVID-19 in young people. International Journal of Environmental Research and Public Health, 19; 5004.

Kim DS, Kim HS, Scwartz-Barcott D, Zuckett D. (2006). The nature of hope in hospitalized chronically ill patients. International Journal of Nursing Studies, 43; 547–556.

Kortte KB, Wegener ST. (2004). Denial of illness in medical rehabilitation populations: Theory, research and definition. Rehabilitation Psychology, 49; 187–199.

Kralik D, Koch T, Price K, Howard N. (2004). Chronic illness self-management: Taking action to create order. Journal of Clinical Nursing, 13; 259–267.

Kylmä J, Turunen H, Perälä M-L. (1996). Hope and chronic illness: The meaning of hope and ways of fostering hope experienced by chronically ill finish people. International Journal of Nursing Practice, 2; 209–214.

Kylmä J, Vehviläinen-Julkunen K. (1997). Hope in nursing research: A meta-analysis of the ontological and epistemological foundations of research on hope. Journal of Advanced Nursing, 25; 211–427.

Lacerda EM, McDermott C, Kingdon CC, Butterworth J, Cliff JM, Nacul L. (2019). Hope, disappointment and perseverance: Reflections of people with Myalgic encephalomyelitis/chronic fatigue syndrome (ME/CFS) and multiple sclerosis participating in biomedical research. A qualitative focus group study. Health Expectations, 22; 373–384.

Laranjeira, C., Querido, A. (2022). Hope and optimism as an opportynity to improve the "postive mental health" demand. Frontiers in Psychology, 13: 827320. DOI:https://doi.org/10.3389%2Ffpsyg.2022.827320

Laskiwski S, Morse JM. (1993). The patient with spinal cord injury: The modification of hope and expressions of despair. Canadian Journal of Rehabilitation, 6(3); 143–153.

Lazarus RS. (1966). Psychological stress and the coping process. New York: McGraw-Hill.

Lazarus RS. (1999). Hope: An emotion and vital coping resource against despair. Social Research, 66; 653–678.

Lazarus RS, Folkman S. (1984). Stress, appraisal, and coping. New York: Springer.

Leite ACAB, García-Vivar C, DeMontigny F, Nascimento LC. (2021). Waves of family hope: Narratives of families in the context of paediatric chronic illness. Revista Latino-Americana de Enfermagem, 29; e3504.

Lennings CJ. (1996). Self-efficacy and temporal orientation as predictors of treatment outcome in severely dependent alcoholics. Alcoholism Treatment Quarterly, 14; 71–79.

Leverson RW. (1994). Human emotion: A functional view. In P Ekman & RJ Davidson (Eds.), The nature of emotion: Fundamental questions (pp. 123–126). Oxford: Oxford University Press.

Leverson RW, Gottman JM. (1983). Marital interaction: Physiological linkage and affective exchange. Journal of Personality and Social Psychology, 45; 587–597.

Lewin K. (1951). Field theory in social science. New York: Harper.

Livneh H. (2009). Denial of chronic illness and disability: Part 1. Theoretical, functional, and dynamic perspectives. *Rehabilitation Counseling Bulletin*, 52(4); 225–236. https://doi.org/10.1177/0034355209333689

Livneh H. (2012). The concept of time in rehabilitation and psychosocial adaptation to chronic illness and disability: Part I. Rehabilitation Counseling Bulletin, 55(4); 195–206.

Livneh H. (2013). The concept of time in rehabilitation and psychosocial adaptation to chronic illness and disability: Part II. Rehabilitation Counseling Bulletin, 56(2); 71–84.

Livneh H. (2015). Quality of life and coping with chronic illness and disability: A temporal perspective. Rehabilitation Counseling Bulletin, 59; 67–83.

Livneh H. (2022). Can the concepts of energy and psychological energy enrich our understanding of psychosocial adaptation to traumatic experiences, chronic illnesses, and disabilities. Frontiers in Psychology, 13; 1–18.

Locke J. (1975). An essay concerning human understanding (Bk II, Ch XX). Edited by P Nidditch. Oxford: Clarendon.

Lohne V, Severinsson E. (2004). Hope during the first months after acute spinal cord injury. Journal of Advanced Nursing, 47; 1–9.

Long KNG, Kim ES, Chen Y, Wilson MF, Worthington EL, VanderWeele TJ. (2020). The role of hope in subsequent health and well-being for older adults: An outcome-wide longitudinal approach. Global Epidemiology, 2; 100018.

Lynch WF. (1965). Images of hope: Imagination as healer of the hopeless. Baltimore, MD: Helicon.

Mairami FF, Warren N, Allotey PA, Reidpath DD. (2020). Contextual factors that shape recovery after stroke in Malaysia, Disability and Rehabilitation, 42; 3189–3198.

Marcel, G. (1951). Homo Viator: Introduction to a metaphysics of hope (pp. 29–31) (E. Crawford, Trans.). Chicago: Henry Regnery.

Marques, S.C., Lopez, S.J. (2017). The Development of Hope. In: Wehmeyer, M., Shogren, K., Little, T., Lopez, S. (eds) Development of Self-Determination Through the Life-Course. Springer, Dordrecht. https://doi.org/10.1007/978-94-024-1042-6_21

Mazanderani F, Kelly J, Ducey A. (2017). From embodied risk to embodying hope: Therapeutic experimentation and experiential information sharing in a contest intervention for multiple Sclerosis. BioSocieties, 13; 232–254.

Mazanderani F, Hughes N, Hardy C, Sillence E, Powell, J. (2019). Health information work and the enactment of care in couples and families affected by Multiple Sclerosis. *Sociology of Health and Illness*, 41; 385–410. DOI: https://doi.org/10.1111/1467-9566.12842

McAdams DP, Guo J. (2015). Narrating the generative life. Psychological Science, 26; 475–483.

McAdams DP, Reynolds J, Lewis M, Patten AH, Bowman PJ. (2001). When bad things turn good and good things turn bad: Sequences of redemption and contamination in life narrative and their relation to psychosocial adaptation in midlife adults and in students. Personality and Social Psychology Bulletin, 27; 387–505.

McCracken LM, Vowles KE, Eccleston C. (2004). Acceptance of chronic pain: Component analysis and a revised assessment method. Pain, 107; 159–166.

Menninger K. (1959). The academic lecture: Hope. The *American Journal of Psychiatry*, 116; 481–491. https://doi.org/10.1176/ajp.116.6.481

Miller EK. (2000). The prefrontal cortex and cognitive control. Nature Reviews in Neuroscience. 1; 59–65.

Miller JF. (1991). Developing and maintaining hope in families of the critically ill. AACN Clinical Issues in Critical Care Nursing, 2; 307–365.

Miller JF. (2007). Hope: A construct central to nursing. Nursing Forum, 42; 1–46.

Miller WR, Rollnick S. (2013). Motivational interviewing: Preparing people for change (3rd ed.). New York: Guildford Press.

Mishel MH. (1988). Uncertainty in illness. Image: Journal of Nursing Scholarship, 4; 225–232.

Mishel MH. (1990). Reconceptualization of the uncertainty in illness theory. Image: Journal of Nursing Scholarship, 22; 256–262.

Momen N, Hadfield P, Kuhn I, Smith E, Barclay S. (2012). Discussing an uncertain future: End-of-life care conversations in chronic obstructive pulmonary disease. A systematic literature review and narrative synthesis. Thorax, 1–4.

Morse JM, Doberneck B. (1995). Delineating the concept of hope. Image, 27; 277–285.

Moss B, Northcott S, Behn N, Monnelly K, Marshall J, Thomas S, Simpson A, Goldsmith K, McVicker S, Flood C, Hilari K. (2021). 'Emotion is of the essence . . . number on priority': A nested qualitative study exploring psychosocial adjustment to stroke and aphasia. International Journal of Language and Communication Disorders, 56; 594–608.

Murphy ER. (2023). Hope and well-being. Current Opinion in Psychology, 50; 101558.

Nekolaichuk CL. (1999). The meaning of hope in health and illness. Bioethics Forum, 15(1); 14–20.

Nell W, Rothmann S. (2018). Hope: Religiosity, and subjective well-being. Journal of Psychology Africa, 28; 253–260.

Nowotny M. (1989). Assessment of hope in patients with cancer: Development of an instrument. Oncology Nursing Forum, 16(1); 57–61.

Oettingen G, Gollwitzer PM. (2002). Turning hope thoughts into goal-directed behaviour. Psychological Inquiry, 13; 304–307.

Owen D. (1989). Nurse's perspective on the meaning of hope in patients with cancer: A qualitative study. Oncology Nursing Forum, 16; 75–79.

Parker-Oliver D. (2002). Redefining hope for the terminally ill. American Journal of Hospice and Palliative Care, 19; 115–120.

Patiero C, Fava GA, Carrozzino D. (2023). Illness denial in medical disorders: A systematic review. Systematic Review, 92; 211–226.

Penz K, Duggleby W. (2011). Harmonizing hope: A grounded theory study of the experience of hope of registered nurses who provide palliative care in community settings. Palliative and Supportive Care, 9; 281–294.

Pinsent A. (2020). Chapter 3. Hope as a virtue in the middle ages. In SC an den Heuvel (Ed.), Historical and multidisciplinary perspectives on hope (pp. 47–60).

Pinto MH, Andrade AC, Leite B, Rhibna R, Kusmusmota L. (2023). Experience of hope in older people with chronic illness: A meta synthesis. International Journal of Older People Nursing, 19; e12579.

Pleeging E, Burger M, Exel JV. (2021). The relations between hope and subjective well-being: A literature overview and empirical analysis. Applied Research in Quality of Life, 16: 1019–1041.

Posner J, Russell JA, Peterson BS. (2005). The circumplex model of affect: An integrative approach to affective neuroscience, cognitive development, and psychopathology. Developments in Psychopathology, 17; 715–734.

Pruyser, W. (1986). Maintaining hope in adversity. Pastoral Psychology, 35; 120–131.

Qama, E, Diviani, N., Grignoli, N., Rubinelli, S. (2022). Health professionals' view on the role of hope and communication challenges with patients in palliative care: A systematic narrative review, Patient Education and Counseling, 105; 1470–1487. https://doi.org/10.1016/j.pec.2021.09.025.:

Rabinowitz T, Peirson R. (2006). "Nothing is wrong, doctor": Understanding and managing denial in patients with cancer. Cancer Investigation, 24; 68–76.

Rand KL. (2018). Hope, self-efficacy, and optimism: Conceptual and empirical differences. In MW Gallagher & SJ Lopez (Eds.), The Oxford book of hope (pp. 45–58). Oxford: Oxford University Press.

Reder EAK, Serwint JR. (2009). Unti the last breath. Exploring the concept of hope for parents and health care professionals during a child's serious illness. Archives of Paediatric and Adolescent Medicine, 163; 653–657.

Reynolds F, Prior S. (2003). Sticking jewels in your life: Exploring women's strategies for negotiating an acceptable quality of life with multiple sclerosis. Qualitative Health Research, 13, 1225–1251.

Robichaud C, Simpson C. (2013). Finding a place for hope in the management of chronic illness. Dalhousie Medical Journal, 40; 33–35.

Rosenberg A, Arnold RM, Schenker Y. (2021). Holding hope for patients with serious illness. Journal of the American Medical Association, 326; 1259–1260.

Russell JA. (1980). A circumplex model of affect. Journal of Personality and Social Psychology, 39; 1161.

Sælør KT, Ness O, Holgersen H, Davidson L. (2014). Hope and recovery: A scoping review. Advances in Dual Diagnosis, 7; 63–72.

Safri T. (2016). Hope: A psychological perspective. Indian Journal of Positive Psychology, 7; 138–140.

Scobbie L, Thomson K, Pollock A, Evans J. Goal adjustment by people living with long-term conditions: A scoping review of literature published from January 2007 to June 2018. Neuropsychol Rehabil. 2021 Sep;31(8); 1314–1345. doi: 10.1080/09602011.2020.1774397. Epub 2020 Jun 11. PMID: 32525446.

Schmidt JE, Andrykowski MA. (2004). The role of social and dispositional variables associated with emotional processing in adjustment to breast cancer: An internet-based study. Health Psychology, 23; 259–266. https://doi.org/10.1037/0278-6133.23.3.259

Schrank B, Woppmann A, Sibitz I, Lauber C. (2010). Development and validation of an integrative scale to assess hope. Health Expect. 2011 Dec;14(4):417–28. doi: 10.1111/j.1369-7625.2010.00645.x.

Scioli A, Ricci M, Nyugen T, Scioli RR. (2011). Hope: Its nature and measurement. Psychology of Religion and Spirituality, 3; 78–97.

Simpson C. (2004). When hope makes us vulnerable: A discussion of patient-healthcare provider interactions in the context of hope. Bioethics, 18; 428–447.

Smedema SM, Bakken-Gillen SK, Dalton J. (2009). Psychosocial adaptation to chronic illness and disability: Models and measurement. In F Chang, E da Silva Cardoso, & JA Chronister (Eds.), Understanding psychosocial adjustment to chronic illness and disability (pp. 51–73). New York: Springer.

Smith NH. (2008). Analysing hope. Critical Horizons: A Journal of Philosophy and Social Theory, 9(1); 5–23.

Snyder CR, Harris C, Anderson JR, Holleran SA, Irving LM, Sigmon ST, Yoshinobu L, Gibb J, Langelle C, Harney P. (1991). The will and the ways: development and validation of an individual-differences measure of hope. Journal of Personality and Social Psycholgy, 60(4):570–85. doi: 10.1037//0022-3514.60.4.570.

Snyder CR, Irving LM, Anderson JR. (1991). Hope and health. Handbook of Social and Clinical Psychology: The Health Perspective, 162; 285–305.

Snyder, C. R. (2002). Hope theory: Rainbows in the mind. Psychological Inquiry, 13(4), 249–275. https://doi.org/10.1207/S15327965PLI1304_01

Snyder CR, Rand KL, King EA, Feldman DB, Woodward JT. (2002). "False" hope. Journal of Clinical Psychology, 58; 1003–1022. https://doi.org/10.1002/jclp.10096

Soundy A, Benson J, Dawes H, Smith B, Collett J, Meaney A. (2012) Understanding hope in patients with Multiple Sclerosis. Physiotherapy. 98(4); 344–350. doi: 10.1016/j.physio.2011.05.003. Epub 2011 Jun 17. PMID: 23122442.

Soundy, A., Smith, B., Dawes, H., Pall, H., Gimbrere, K., & Ramsay, J. (2013). Patient's expression of hope and illness narratives in three neurological conditions: a meta-ethnography. Health Psychology Review, 7(2), 177–201. https://doi.org/10.1080/17437199.2011.568856

Soundy A. (2018) Psycho-emotional content of illness narrative master plots for people with chronic illness: Implications for assessment. World Journal of Psychiatry, 20;8:79–82.

Soundy A, Condon C. (2015). Patients' experiences of maintaining mental well-being and hope within motor neuron disease: A thematic synthesis. Frontiers in Psychology, 6; 606.

Soundy A, Forkner A, Bresloff A, Palser H, Bamford T, Mrowiec D, Reed A, Chan C. (2023). Testing a psychological tool to enhance hope in people with stroke; A qualitative study. Preprints, 2023101319. https://doi.org/10.20944/preprints202310.1319.v2

Soundy A, Hemmings L, Gardiner L, Rosewilliam S, Heneghan NR, Cronin K, Reid K. (2021b). E-learning communication skills training for physiotherapy students: A two phased sequential mixed methods study. Patient Education and Counseling, 104; 2045–2053.

Soundy A, Liles C, Stubbs B, Roskell C. (2014b). Identifying a framework of hope in order to establish the importance of generalised hopes for individuals who have suffered a stroke. Advances in Medicine, 471874.

Soundy A, Mohan V, Room J, Morris J, Fazakarley L, Stiger R. (2024). Psychological skills training using simulated practice for brief therapeutic interactions. International Journal of Healthcare Simulation, 1–14. https://doi.org/10.54531/sdaz6915

Soundy A, Rosenbaum S, Elder T, Kyte D, Stubbs B, Hemmings L, Roskell C, Collett J, Dawes H. (2016b). The Hope and Adaptation Scale (HAS): Establishing face and content validity. Open Journal of Therapy and Rehabilitation, 4; 76–86.

Soundy A, Roskell C, Elder T, Collett J, Dawes H. (2016a). The psychological processes of adaptation and hope in patients with multiple sclerosis: A thematic synthesis. Open Journal of Therapy and Rehabilitation, 14; 22–47.

Soundy A, Roskell C, Stubbs B, Collett J, Dawes H, Smith B. (2014d). Do you hear what your patient is telling you? Understanding the meaning behind the narrative. Way Ahead, 18; 10–13.

Soundy A, Smith B, Cressy F, Webb L. (2010). The experience of spinal cord injury: Using Frank's narrative types to enhance physiotherapy undergraduates' understanding. Physiotherapy, 96; 52–58.

Soundy A, Stubbs, B, Freeman P, Coffee C, Roskell C. (2014c). Factors influencing patients' hope in stroke and spinal cord injury: A narrative review. International Journal of Therapy and Rehabilitation, 21; 207–246.

Soundy A, Stubbs B, Roskell C. (2014a). The experience of Parkinson's disease: A systematic review and meta-ethnography. Scientific World Journal, 613592.

Stanislawski K. (2019). The coping circumplex model: An integrative model of the structure of coping with stress. Hypothesis and Theory, 10; 694.

Stephenson, C. (1991). The concept of hope revisited for nursing. Journal of Advanced Nursing, 16; 1456–1461. https://doi.org/10.1111/j.1365-2648.1991.tb01593.x

Stempsey WE. (2015). Hope for health and health care. Medical Health Care and Philosophy, 18; 41–49.

Stephenson C. (1991). The concept of hope revisited for nursing. Journal of Advanced Nursing, 16; 1456–1461. https://doi.org/10.1111/j.1365-2648.1991.tb01593.x

Stotland E. (1969). The psychology of hope. Jossey-Bass, San Francisco, USA.

Sturgeon JA, Zautra AJ. (2013). Psychological resilience, pain catastrophising, and positive emotions: Perspectives on comprehensive modelling of individual pain adaptation. Current Pain and Headache Reports, 17; 317.

Subramanian I, Pushparatnam K, McDaniels B, Mathur S, Post B, Schrag A. (2024). Delivering the diagnosis of Parkinson's disease setting the stage with hope and compassion. Parkinsonism and Related Disorders, 118; 105926.

Snyder, C. R. (2002). Hope theory: Rainbows in the mind. Psychological Inquiry, 13(4), 249–275. https://doi.org/10.1207/S15327965PLI1304_01

Synder J, Adams, K, Crooks VA, Whitehurst D, Vallee J. (2014). "I knew what was going to happen if I did nothing and so I was going to do something": Faith, hope and trust in the decisions of Canadians with Multiple Sclerosis to seek unproven interventions abroad. BMC Health Services Research, 14; 445.

Sällfors C, Fasth A, Hallberg LRM. (2002). Oscillating between hope and despair. Child: Care, Health and Development, 28; 495–505.

Taylor SE. (1983). Adjustment to threatening events: A theory of cognitive adaptation. American Psychologist, 38; 1161–1173.

Toye F, Barker K. (2012). 'I can't see any reason for stopping doing anything, but I might have to do it differently' – restoring hope to patients with persistent non-specific low back pain – a qualitative study. Disability and Rehabilitation, 34; 894–903.

Tutton E, Seers K, Langstaff D. (2009). An exploration of hope as a concept for nursing. Journal of Orthopaedic Nursing, 13; 119–127.

Ursin H, Eriksen HR. (2003). The cognitive activation theory of stress. Psychoneuroendrocrinology, 39; 567–592.

Venning A, Eliott J, Wilson A, Kettler L. (2008). Understanding young peoples' experience of chronic illness: A systematic review. International Journal of Evidence Based Healthcare, 6; 321–336.

Weis R, Speridkos EC. (2011). A meta-analysis of hope enhancement strategies in clinical and community settings. Psychology of Well-Being: Theory, Research and Practice, 1; 5.

Wigfield A, & Eccles JS. (2000). Expectancy–value theory of achievement motivation. Contemporary Educational Psychology, 25(1); 68–81. https://doi.org/10.1006/ceps.1999.1015. PMID: 10620382.

Wiles R, Cott C, Gibson BE. (2008). Hope, expectations, and recovery from illness: A narrative synthesis of qualitative research. Journal of Advanced Nursing, 54; 564–573.

Wright BA. (1983). Physical disability-a psychosocial approach (2nd ed.). New York: Harper and Row.

Ziebland S, Renata, K. (2012). Metaphoric language and the articulation of emotions by people affected by motor neurone disease. Chronic Illness, 8; 159–236.

Zimbardo PG, Boyd JN. (1999). Putting time in perspective: A valid, reliable individual-differences metric. Journal of Personality and Social Psychology, 77; 1271–1288.

Index

For Product Safety Concerns and Information please contact our EU
representative GPSR@taylorandfrancis.com Taylor & Francis Verlag GmbH,
Kaufingerstraße 24, 80331 München, Germany

Printed and bound by CPI Group (UK) Ltd, Croydon, CR0 4YY
11/06/2025
01899269-0001

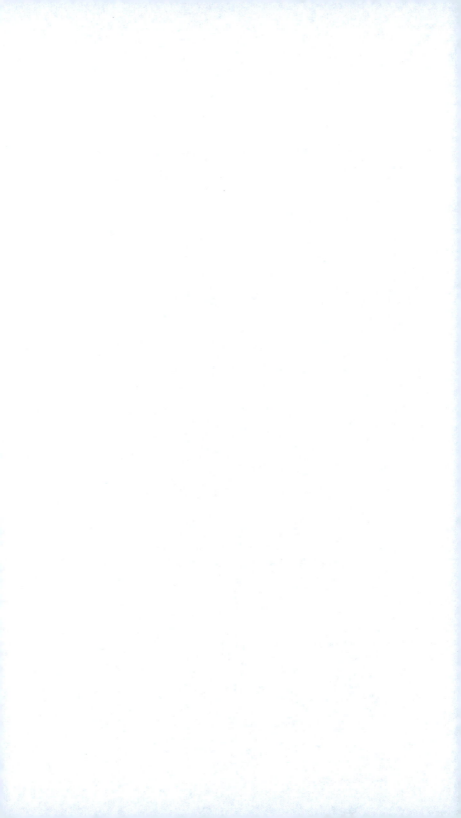